the intuitive
eating *plan*

the **intuitive eating** *plan*

A Body-Positive Approach
to Rebuilding Your Relationship with Food

**ROCKRIDGE
PRESS**

Kirsten Ackerman, MS, RD

For general information on our other products and services or to obtain technical support, please contact our Customer Care Department within the United States at (866) 744-2665, or outside the United States at (510) 253-0500.

Rockridge Press publishes its books in a variety of electronic and print formats. Some content that appears in print may not be available in electronic books, and vice versa.

Interior and Cover Designer: Gabe Nansen
Art Producer: Sue Bischofberger
Editor: Marisa A. Hines and Shabnam Sigman
Production Manager: Michael Kay
Production Editors: Sigi Nacson and Andrew Yackira

ISBN: Print 978-1-64611-788-8 | eBook 978-1-64611-789-5
R0

For my mom, who has accompanied me on this journey in many ways, and for my dad, who has always encouraged me to "subvert the dominant paradigm."

Contents

Introduction

I first learned about Intuitive Eating through the *Food Psych* podcast, hosted by a fellow Anti-Diet Dietitian, Christy Harrison. At the time, I had two degrees in nutrition and a certification as a Registered Dietitian, and I had been working in the field for about a year, providing nutrition counseling under the traditional weight-centric model.

Up until that time, I never would have identified as a dieter. Dieting was something my mother did throughout my childhood on her various stints with NutriSystem and Weight Watchers. It was not something I thought of engaging in. In fact, as I unknowingly struggled with disordered eating throughout my late teens and early adulthood, I ironically held a firm belief that diets did not work. Upon learning about Intuitive Eating, my eyes finally opened to all of the ways in which the diet mentality had long been infecting my relationship with food.

With the support of a growing Intuitive Eating community, I became curious about the guilt and shame I felt around my food preferences and behaviors. I began to question my long-held beliefs about body size and health. I became curious about my inclinations to hide candy wrappers under paper towels in the trash can and bend the truth about how often I ate fast food. I challenged the notion that obsessively tracking calories in

MyFitnessPal for the purpose of controlling my body size was a normal, responsible behavior.

Upon further inspection, I realized that the diet mentality was rampant in my life. I was living in a state of restriction, deprivation, and obsession with food and body image that was wrapped in a cloak of perfectly posed gym selfies. Friends, family, and acquaintances praised my behavior. They were in awe of my dedication and consistency. I received envious compliments on my shrinking body, even as my inner world was reduced to nothing but thoughts of food, body, and exercise.

When I learned about Intuitive Eating, an irrevocable shift occurred. In many ways, relief set in. I wasn't lacking willpower or the necessary motivation to properly maintain the weight loss I achieved for small periods of time. It wasn't that I just hadn't found the right diet yet. No, it wasn't *me* at all. It was the entire *culture* that was the problem. And yet, learning about Intuitive Eating also marked the beginning of a period of time when I felt a bit lost. The blinders had been taken off, and now, everywhere I looked, I saw Diet Culture's harmful messaging. It is not easy to feel alone in knowing such a disruptive truth.

One of the most common struggles I hear about from clients on their Intuitive Eating journey is that they feel unsure of how to apply the principles in their lives. It is common to feel lost in the early stages of Intuitive Eating, because we are used to having the clearly outlined, rigid, external guidance of a diet plan (or the glittery version of a "lifestyle change"). Rules feel safe and can meet an unmet need within us for a sense of control. Whereas diets provide solid—albeit suffocating—rules, Intuitive Eating brings you back to the wisdom of your body, which is inherently a bit less black and white.

Embracing Intuitive Eating may involve peeling back some of the layers behind a need to control. However, the desire for structure on your journey is understandable. In fact, I see the entire framework of Intuitive Eating as a bridge from the suffocating structure of dieting to the freedom of being in sync with your body. Giving up the diet mentality is a process, a journey. It is not a shift made overnight. If you feel unsure of how to apply these principles, or of how you can honor your health in a way that is free of diet mentality, this book is for you.

As an Anti-Diet Registered Dietitian and Certified Intuitive Eating Counselor with my own personal experience recovering from disordered eating, I am equipped with the knowledge to guide you through the steps necessary to heal your relationship with food. I work daily with clients who are struggling along the disordered eating spectrum, and my passion for this topic is born out of the very real pain I endured from my struggles and from the very real liberation I found on my recovery journey.

My hope is that, as you read this book, you will feel supported and gently guided back toward yourself. It will be uncomfortable. It will be challenging. But on the other side is not only a healed relationship with food, but also a healed relationship with yourself that is guaranteed to impact every area of your life.

Getting the Most Out of This Book

This book will provide direction for you to begin experiencing life in a new way. Healing your relationship with food through Intuitive Eating is not just about the food. It is much more about the things you have more time for when food does not hold such a chaotic role in your life. When you are fixated on food and body, your brain space is consumed with thoughts of recipes, calories, macronutrients, workouts, and unfulfilled cravings. When you take healing steps away from food and body fixation, you are more able to be present in your life with the things that truly matter. Welcome to your guide away from fixation and toward freedom.

Practice Is Key

Be gentle with yourself during this process. Learning to eat and relate to food and your body in a new way is challenging. This new way of thinking and eating defies the cultural norm. You may find you have been following certain food rules for so long that you do not even remember where you learned them. You may find yourself strangely attached to and defensive of certain food rules. Continue to lead with curiosity. You will likely become painfully aware of the many ways you have become accustomed to relying on external guidance for choosing food rather than the wisdom of your own body.

In this book, you will be introduced to concepts that challenge what you previously knew about food, bodies, and wellness. You will be introduced to the principles of Intuitive Eating, as well as exercises that will allow you to dive in and do the work for yourself. As you move through the book, I encourage you to go back to previous chapters and repeat the exercises. Returning to these ideas, learning to reframe previously held beliefs, and practicing new skills are key to this journey. Intuitive Eating is a process that requires time and continued curiosity.

Journaling is often a helpful step during the healing process to support uncovering the deeper layers behind your behaviors. The journal can be a space to practice, repeat, and explore the exercises introduced in this book. If a particular exercise feels triggering, consider that feeling to be your invitation to put it on the back burner. Keeping a journal during this process to practice new skills and exercises is meant to support your reconnection to your body. If an exercise does not feel supportive, come back to it another time.

There's No Way to Fail

Reconnecting to your body through the framework of Intuitive Eating is not a pass or fail endeavor. Diet Culture says you are either on track or off track, on the wagon or off the wagon, succeeding or failing. In other words, it sets you up to fail. It does not allow you to be human. Consider Intuitive Eating your permission to be messy. Embracing messiness is how we learn, how we grow, and how we become a version of ourselves that feels more authentic and aligned.

This experience will surely be filled with moments when you feel disconnected from your body. There will be times when you find yourself eating mindlessly, urgently, or chaotically. There will be times when you eat past a comfortable state of fullness or times when you feel enticed by the promise of a new diet. In these moments, choose curiosity and compassion. The principles of Intuitive Eating are not rules. They cannot be broken. They are meant to be a guide for you to understand uncomfortable patterns and harmful beliefs about food and your body so that you can illuminate a path forward that is more supportive.

Witnessing disordered behaviors around food during this process is not a sign of failure. It is an expected and welcomed part of this learning process. It is an opportunity for growth and understanding. And once you adopt a mind-set of curiosity, each experience will provide you with information that will strengthen your relationships with food and your body.

Vision Exercise

Dieting consumes a lot of time and energy. It makes it difficult to explore who we are and what we value.

For this exercise, reflect on what you hope to gain from this book.

What is your vision for your future relationship with food?

What do you hope to gain more time for when you spend less time consumed by thoughts about food and body?

You've Got This

If your hope is that you will find more connection to your body and more peace in your choices around food, you are on the right path. Remember, this book will serve as your guide back to yourself and the life that you want to live. It is difficult to feel passionate and have clarity in your life when your mind is fogged up by an obsession with food and body.

This book will help you understand the culture around you and how it has impacted your relationship with food and your body. In the chapters that follow, you will learn how to reconnect to your body's wisdom so you don't need to live with fear and a fixation around food. If you have read up to this point, trust that this book is for you and you are ready to do the work.

Chapter One

Eating Intuitively

Intuitive Eating is an evidence-based framework developed by two registered dietitians, Evelyn Tribole and Elyse Resch. In this chapter, we will cover an overview of the 10 principles of Intuitive Eating. We will also review additional resources and information about eating disorders. The approach has recently gained momentum, likely due to the fact that people are catching on to the pitfalls of Diet Culture. The jig is up. We have come to realize the ways that dieting has done us wrong. Diets have not delivered on making us healthier, happier, or smaller; they have only led us down a path of food and body fixation.

The principles outlined in this chapter are meant to be used as a framework for fostering a new relationship with food and your body. Some of the principles involve mental shifts around the way you view food, your body and movement, and the beliefs you hold around them. Some of the principles will require physical shifts, such as increasing awareness around body cues like hunger and fullness. And other principles will illuminate the ways in which emotions can impact your behavior around food. Each of the principles will serve to reconnect you to your body so you can reclaim your role as the expert of your own body.

Intuitive Eating: Core Principles

With the increase in popularity of Intuitive Eating, there has also been an increase in misinterpretations of the approach. One of the most common and most harmful misinterpretations is that Intuitive Eating is a diet or a weight loss method. This is in direct contrast to the core philosophies behind Intuitive Eating, which are weight inclusivity, Health at Every Size, and anti-diet nutrition. There is no weight goal associated with Intuitive Eating. In this way, it is weight neutral.

Intuitive Eating is also not anti-weight loss. Weight may increase, decrease, or stay the same when practicing Intuitive Eating. The result is not a measurement of progress or failure, because *weight is not the focus.*

Another misconception of Intuitive Eating is that it is anti-health or anti-nutrition. In reality, Intuitive Eating is designed to alleviate the disconnection between our bodies and the food we eat, which can often cause chaotic, dissatisfying eating. This state of eating impacts both our health and our nutrition in negative ways.

Intuitive Eating doesn't necessarily mean eating whatever you want, whenever you want. Attunement to your body's cues enables you to understand and honor your own needs more effectively. It is worth noting that there is nothing morally wrong with eating whatever you want, whenever you want. In fact, doing so is often a necessary step in healing from dieting after a long period of not being able to seek satisfaction in eating. That is perfectly okay. You have permission to allow your process to unfold.

PRINCIPLE 1: Reject the Diet Mentality

The diet mentality is a state of mind. Yes, following a diet plan is problematic. But, in the modern day, the diet mentality is much sneakier than that. It does not necessarily need to be accompanied by a structured plan, but rather could be an assortment of rigid rules regarded as a "lifestyle change."

- A telltale sign of diet mentality is the feeling of either being "on track" or "off track." If there is a wagon to fall off of, it's diet mentality.

- Another key element of diet mentality is the reliance on external sources to guide eating choices (Tribole and Resch 2012). Rather than tuning in to the wisdom of your own body, you follow an external rule of what, when, or how much you believe you should eat.

- Finally, diet mentality is characterized by a focus on weight or weight loss. A weight loss focus inherently disconnects us from our bodies. When weight loss is the focus, decreasing the number on the scale takes priority over adequately nourishing ourselves and honoring our bodies' cues.

An essential aspect of Intuitive Eating is a commitment to reject the diet mentality and replace it with awareness, curiosity, and attunement to your own body's cues. You will be guided through exercises in the book to support these shifts.

PRINCIPLE 2: Honor Your Hunger

One of the hallmarks of diet mentality is ignoring or attempting to suppress hunger. Somehow, Diet Culture has convinced us that it is healthy to disregard one of the most basic and life-sustaining cues of our bodies.

When you suppress your body's hunger cues, physiology always wins. A stick of gum or a cup of coffee may keep hunger at bay for a while, but your body responds with proportionally increased and chaotic cravings when the hunger returns. It may drive you to seek high-calorie, carbohydrate-rich foods later that night in an attempt to overcompensate for the earlier deprivation. It is likely that at times like this, you will blame yourself for not being able to control yourself, or assume that you have an unnatural affinity for these foods. But the reality is that it is your disconnection from your body that is fueling the chaos. Your body is trying to save you from being deprived of an essential element for sustaining life: food. You are deserving of nourishment.

There are a few key elements to honoring hunger:

- Realizing you deserve adequate nourishment
- Realizing adequate nourishment is healthy
- Becoming attuned to and aware of your body's cues
- Having the food available when hunger arises

PRINCIPLE 3: Make Peace with Food

There is no moral value to food choices (Tribole and Resch 2012). You are not good for eating a salad or bad for having dessert. Practice full permission to eat all foods. The irony of trying to avoid or cut out certain foods is that doing so drives cravings for those foods. We want what we cannot have. When it comes to biology and basic life needs (air, water, food), we become obsessed with what we sense is scarce. If we cut out chocolate, our body drives us to seek out chocolate.

We think about it nonstop. We obsess over it until we have it. And then, when we finally have it, we have it in excess to overcompensate for the feeling of scarcity. This response is natural and protective.

Making peace with food eliminates a source of chaos in our relationship with food. Rather than oscillating from feeling deprived and obsessed to feeling overindulged and ashamed, we open ourselves up to feeling satisfied, content, and peaceful around food.

A common hesitation people have about exploring full permission to eat is the thought that doing so will lead to eating large quantities of highly feared foods. When you first reintroduce previously restricted foods, the pendulum may swing to the other side: overeating. This is your body's natural reaction to restriction. However, over time, that reaction will subside and settle down in the absence of restrictive behaviors and the diet mentality.

The point of making peace with food is not to eat less or lose weight. The point is to lead you to the relationship with food that you deserve: a comfortable, satisfying, pleasurable one that is not spoiled by harmful beliefs about it.

PRINCIPLE 4: Challenge the Food Police

The food police are a compilation of all the food rules you have subscribed to over the years (Tribole and Resch 2012). Food rules are based on external sources of information and are often not aligned with your personal experience in your body. Food rules are also very black and white.

An important piece of returning to Intuitive Eating is questioning these long-held, deeply rooted beliefs. Examples of food police thoughts may be *"I should never eat after 8 p.m.," "I should only buy food from the perimeter of the grocery store,"* or *"I should not eat any added sugar."* Although sometimes seemingly health promoting, food police thoughts keep us rooted in diet mentality and disconnected from our bodies, a state which is ultimately detrimental to our health. Call out food police thoughts when you notice them so you can start to untangle your attachments to them (Tribole and Resch 2012).

PRINCIPLE 5: Feel Your Fullness

Become curious about the different sensations associated with fullness in your body. Experiencing different levels of fullness is normal. We can gain a lot of information when we get curious about the variables that lead to eating past fullness or not eating enough to meet our needs.

When you notice you eat past fullness at dinner, the first response may be a sense of failure. That is understandable, considering we live in a culture that encourages us to eat the least amount physically possible. But if you allow yourself to peel back another layer from that experience, you may find that you had not eaten in many hours and were ravenous. You may have been disconnected from your hunger cues for so long that you did not even recognize or think to consider your hunger level. These types of revelations will go a long way in helping you to figure out how to best meet your body's needs and to arrive at a place where eating to comfortable fullness is the norm (although not a rule).

Full permission to eat is a very important prerequisite to being able to trust your body to stop eating at a comfortable place of fullness (Tribole and Resch 2012). For instance, perhaps you are limiting or monitoring your intake of ice cream and find yourself eating past a comfortable place of fullness every time you allow yourself to eat it. The likely reason is that your body feels an urgency to get it all in right now, knowing that you will not allow that food later. Adequate and consistent nourishment throughout the day also plays a key role in your ability to stop at a comfortable state of fullness.

PRINCIPLE 6: Discover the Satisfaction Factor

Satisfaction is an often overlooked element in eating that plays an important role in our behavior around food. Allow yourself to find pleasure in your eating experiences. Choose foods that sound delicious and satisfying to you in the moment. Bring awareness to what foods and sensory qualities sound appealing. Whereas diet mentality urges you to stick to the plan and follow externally prescribed rules, this principle of

Intuitive Eating encourages you to use the wisdom of your own body's cravings to guide you.

When you eliminate a particular food, you often find yourself with intense cravings for that food. You may try to find another "allowable" food to satisfy that craving. But instead, what usually happens is you end up eating the apple, the cheese stick, the popcorn, the rice cake, only to find yourself face-first in the gallon of ice cream in the end anyway. If you had given yourself permission to use satisfaction as a guide, you would have eaten the ice cream and moved on, which is obviously a more satisfying experience in the end.

PRINCIPLE 7: Cope with Your Emotions with Kindness

There is nothing morally wrong with emotional eating. In fact, emotional eating is a human thing. We eat to celebrate and to connect with each other. And sometimes we eat to soothe.

Keep in mind that the goal is not to eliminate using food as a coping mechanism, but rather to expand your toolbox. Do not feel that you must exclusively choose to either use your old coping skill of emotional eating *or* rely on a new coping skill. Give yourself permission to do both. Fall back on your old, comfortable habit of using food to cope, then intentionally choose to practice another skill as well. In time, the new skill will feel more comforting, and you will have added a skill to your toolbox.

Emotional eating is often demonized in Diet Culture because Diet Culture is obsessed with eating the least amount possible. Emotional eating is a perfectly natural part of being human and does not need to be eradicated in order to heal your relationship with food.

However, there are ways to cope with emotions that may leave you feeling better by addressing what is going on for you in a more direct way. Start tuning in and building awareness around the emotions you are experiencing, especially in moments when you find yourself reaching for food outside of physical hunger (Tribole and Resch 2012). Consider these moments red flags that indicate you are experiencing something on an emotional level that needs tending to. Refrain from purposely avoiding emotional eating in these moments, since doing so is likely to trigger feelings of deprivation.

PRINCIPLE 8: Respect Your Body

Many people fall victim to disordered eating because they are convinced that their body is a problem to be fixed. How could you be convinced otherwise when you live in a culture that sells you that message daily? Healing your relationship to your body is a key underlying element of healing your relationship with food.

Your body is not a problem. Come to terms with the fact that natural body diversity exists (Tribole and Resch 2012; Bacon and Aphramor 2014). In the same way that bodies are diverse in hair color, shoe size, skin color, and height, bodies are diverse in shape and size.

Accept your own genetic blueprint (Tribole and Resch 2012). Consider the ways you can treat your body with more respect and care:

- How can you nourish it in a way that feels supportive?

- How can you honor its cravings in a way that feels satisfying?

- How can you engage in movement in a way that feels good?

- How can you make space for the negative thoughts about your body that you have held on to for so long, while also recognizing the false beliefs that support them?

- How can you express gratitude about what your body does for you?

- How can you channel negative feelings about your body away from yourself and toward the culture that planted these false beliefs?

PRINCIPLE 9: Movement—Feel the Difference

So often in our culture, dieting and weight loss are inextricably linked with movement. When you are "on the wagon," you are dieting and exercising. When you are inevitably "off the wagon," you are not dieting and not exercising. I urge you to find ways of exploring movement that are not motivated by the number of calories it will burn, but rather by how much joy you will experience from it. If you have never found joy in movement or have disabilities that make it difficult to find joy in movement, understand that movement is not a moral obligation. If you choose to engage in movement, allow the movement you choose to be guided by what will serve you best, both physically and mentally.

Movement serves many purposes in our lives:

- It is supportive of both physical and mental health, independent of its impact on body shape or size (Tribole and Resch 2012; Bacon and Aphramor 2011).

- It can serve as a source of pleasure if you are using satisfaction as a guide in choosing types of movement.

- It can be helpful to consider this question: *If you were certain that movement would not have an impact on changing (or maintaining) your body shape or size, what would change about the types of movement you are choosing to engage in?*

It can also be helpful to spend some time considering the types of movement that have been enjoyable to you throughout your life. If you cannot think of any, that is okay, too!

Finally, something Diet Culture diminishes: It is so important to consider rest. Sometimes, the most supportive choice is to skip the walk and choose to watch Netflix on the couch. Health is multifaceted and extends far beyond simply what we eat and how much we move.

PRINCIPLE 10: Honor Your Health—Gentle Nutrition

After spending significant time and energy working to heal your relationships with food and your body, you can start to explore the ways in which adequate nourishment can serve you. It is important to note that this principle can be turned into a diet very easily if interpreted through diet mentality. It is important to do the work of healing your relationships with food and body before working with this principle.

If you find yourself feeling triggered by this principle, skip it for now.

After some time on this journey, you may find yourself in a place where you genuinely want to take steps to support your health through nutrition without falling into the traps of diet mentality.

The most important thing to keep in mind about gentle nutrition is that it is rooted in a mentality of *addition* rather than subtraction. If you are wondering if a particular food practice is aligned with gentle nutrition, ask yourself if it relies on eliminating or cutting back on certain foods. If it does, it is not aligned.

Gentle nutrition is about adding satisfying, nutritious, health-supporting foods to your regular meals. It is also about taking steps to ensure you are getting enough of various nutrients overall, consistently throughout the day. Again, gentle nutrition does not require avoiding, cutting out, or limiting any food at all. It also does not require rigid monitoring or tracking of nutrients. For the vast majority of the population, attempts at rigid manipulation of nutrients are both unnecessary for health and a slippery slope to disordered eating.

Nutrition may not be a priority for everyone on this journey, and that is okay, too. The gentle nutrition principle is here for you if and when it serves you.

Additional Resources for Disordered Eating

Although weight is one of the most common criteria used to diagnose disordered eating, people of all body sizes can suffer from the full range of eating disorders. It is important to recognize that all eating disorders involve restriction of some kind, usually a combination of physical and mental restrictions that can present in different ways.

Examples of common eating disorders include:

Anorexia: An unhealthy disturbance in body image resulting in starvation as well as purging mechanisms of any food that is consumed via self-induced vomiting, laxative use, or extreme exercise

Bulimia: Characterized by episodes of binging (eating an uncomfortable amount of food) followed by purging behaviors

Binge Eating Disorder: Characterized by frequent episodes of eating an uncomfortable amount of food (this type of eating disorder still involves restriction, whether mental, physical, or both)

Other Specified Feeding and Eating Disorder (OSFED): An eating disorder that does not fit within the diagnostic criteria of any of the above disorders, but may engage in many of the same harmful behaviors (Center for Discovery 2020)

>

Avoidant Restrictive Food Intake Disorder (ARFID): Often impacts children and can be misclassified as "picky eating," a disorder characterized by a child being uninterested in eating, having severe aversions to certain tastes or textures of food, or having intense fears around adverse outcomes of eating, such as allergic reaction or choking

Orthorexia: An unhealthy obsession with healthy eating (usually not blatantly motivated by a desire for weight loss; someone with orthorexia is consumed with thoughts of eating the healthiest foods)

If you think you have an eating disorder, it is important that you receive support. These resources may be helpful to you:

- NationalEatingDisorders.org
- CenterForDiscovery.com/blog
- Eating Disorder Screening Tool: NationalEating Disorders.org/screening-tool
- Finding a provider: map.NationalEatingDisorders.org

There are many factors that influence our behaviors and beliefs around food, such as friends, family members, and the culture around us.

Consider the factors that have contributed to your current relationship with food. Remember not to bring judgment into this exercise, only observation and curiosity.

- How did your parents or other role models influence the way you thought about food growing up?

_____

_____

_____

_____

_____

_____

_____

_____

_____

_____

_____

_____

- What have you taken away from different diets you have tried?

_____

_____

_____

_____

_____

_____

_____

- What foods have you learned to fear?

_____

_____

_____

_____

_____

_____

_____

_____

_____

- Has food been a source of comfort for you?

_____

_____

_____

_____

_____

_____

_____

- How might you start to release some of these deep-rooted beliefs about food?

_____

_____

_____

_____

_____

_____

_____

_____

_____

Chapter Two

Food-Positive, Body-Positive

Doing the work to heal your relationships with food and your body is challenging because of the deeply rooted negative beliefs that are reinforced by Diet Culture every day. Diet Culture can be defined as a system of beliefs that prioritizes body shape and body size over true health and well-being (Harrison 2019). More specifically, Diet Culture worships thinness. And it upholds the narrative that weight and health are inextricably linked.

Even recent shifts in popular culture away from weight loss pursuits and toward pursuing health are tainted by the underlying belief that healthier behaviors will result in weight loss.

Diet Culture is a master of eroding the connection between mind and body by convincing us that the expert of our body and our eating is external to ourselves. It is difficult to fully commit to the journey of healing your relationships with food and body if you do not open your eyes to the harmful ways of Diet Culture.

In this chapter, we will cover the essential elements of breaking free from the diet trap, including shifting away from a focus on weight and understanding why restriction backfires. We will also discuss the impact of social media on body image and how to use these digital platforms to your advantage on your journey. Finally, we will cover the roots of the body liberation movement and its evolution, including discussing fat acceptance, body positivity, and the Health at Every Size movement.

Breaking Free from the Diet Trap

According to John LaRosa, President of Marketdata LLC, the diet industry hit a new peak in 2018, growing to 72 billion dollars (LaRosa 2019). The diet industry is essentially a really successful, really profitable scam. It makes us feel insecure about our bodies, and then it preys off the insecurities it creates. From the rebranded WW, formerly Weight Watchers, to Noom (a weight loss app aimed at millennials), bariatric surgery, diet pills, meal replacement shakes, "clean" diet dinner entrées, and medical weight loss, the industry is rampant with solutions that rarely actually work. Yet, the system is designed in such a way that we believe *the diet* worked and it was *us* that failed.

The latest offshoot of Diet Culture is now being recognized as Wellness Culture. Rather than taking a blatant focus on intentional weight loss, this new variation of Diet Culture masks itself as a "healthy lifestyle change." However, the underlying assumption is that weight will be lost as a result of the changes it proposes. Some companies are even co-opting terminology from the anti-diet movement by calling their programs "anti-diets" or "non-diets," and yet they continue to center on weight loss as a goal.

There are two red flags to look out for when assessing whether something is rooted in Diet Culture:

- Restriction (cutting back on or eliminating specific foods)
- Intentional or expected weight loss

Intentional weight loss involves making changes to diet and movement routines specifically for the purpose of achieving weight loss. **Expected weight loss** is the assumption that weight loss is an obvious outcome of adopting healthier behaviors.

Ultimately, dieting does not serve us. It disconnects us from our own bodies and causes harm to the very health it promises to support. And, perhaps most devastating of all, it keeps us from being present in our lives. It's time to find another way.

THE MYTH OF RESTRICTION

Diet Culture tells us we need to cut out, limit, or reduce certain foods. It convinces us that health and happiness are on the other side of food control. Rather than listening to our bodies' cues, we begin to question them and turn to outside sources to guide the food choices we make. With this idea in mind, let's explore two major types of food restriction: physical and mental.

Physical Restriction

When you think of restriction, you likely think of the physical sense of the word: consuming less energy (in the form of calories) than your body requires for normal functioning or cutting out or limiting certain types of food or food groups. This is physical deprivation of the energy your body needs, the satisfaction it craves, or both.

Our bodies are primed to retaliate against restriction (Bacon and Aphramor 2014). Physical restriction sets off a cascade of biological responses, including an increase in hunger, a decrease in satiety (the feeling of fullness and satisfaction after a meal), a decrease in metabolic rate, and an increase in thoughts about food. These biological responses all occur in an evolutionary effort to drive you to seek out food in the presence of a shortage. Whereas Diet Culture encourages us to blame ourselves or (insert unexpected life event here), our biology plays an active role in the "failure" of the diet.

The myth of restriction is that it will result in controlled eating and sustained weight loss. In reality, restriction often results in out-of-control, chaotic eating and, ultimately, weight gain. Of course, Diet Culture would have you believe that these outcomes are due to a lack of willpower, that if you only tried harder or restricted more, it would work. The truth is that these biological responses are virtually insurmountable and protective.

The other type of restriction that can have an equally powerful impact on food behavior is mental restriction.

Mental restriction can show up as a perceived limit or allowable amount of a particular food. Even if you are consuming adequate food for energy, you can experience a sense of food scarcity due to this self-imposed limit. Furthermore, feelings of deprivation can occur if you have experienced true scarcity in your life imposed by dieting from a young age or from a lack of access to food.

Mental deprivation can also result when we are not present for the experience of eating. If you are eating ravenously because you've gone an extended period of time without food, you likely will not be fully present with the sensations or the experience of eating. Therefore, you will not feel satisfied after eating that meal. You will feel mental deprivation despite being physically nourished. And, ultimately, this feeling will drive you to seek out more food.

Mental restriction and deprivation result in many of the same biological responses as physical deprivation. They drive you to seek out food as if there were a physical shortage.

We have long known that restriction leads to chaotic eating. In 1950, a group of researchers published the Minnesota Starvation Study. The study involved male volunteers who spent six months on a semi-starvation diet of about 1,700 calories per day (not far off from many calorie recommendations of diets today). The volunteers developed strange rituals around food. They cut food into small pieces to prolong the enjoyment of the meal, started collecting recipes, and basically became obsessed with food. Some volunteers snuck in food and binged on it. Some had to drop out of the study because of how overwhelmed they became. After the study concluded, likely due to the food deprivation they had experienced, some of the volunteers went on to pursue food-related careers by attending culinary school (Keys, Ancel, Henschel, and Brožek 1950).

The results of this study only confirm what we now know very well: Restriction makes us obsessed with food.

DEVELOPING A POSITIVE RELATIONSHIP WITH FOOD

Food is meant to be pleasurable. It is meant to be a source of joy and connection in our lives. Diet Culture often makes us forget this basic fact. A positive relationship with food is one that provides nourishment, comfort, and satisfaction. It is one that is free of guilt and shame over food choices. It is one in which negative body image thoughts do not impact your behavior around food.

In a positive relationship with food, food is not seen as a means to manipulate the size, shape, or appearance of one's body, but rather a way to provide nourishment and satisfaction. And, finally, a positive relationship with food is one in which body cues are given attention and respected most of the time.

The irony of dieting and intentional weight loss pursuits is that, although they promise to change our behaviors around food and create more control, what they often ultimately do is upset the body's natural balance, which creates a sense of chaos. This outcome impacts behaviors around food. Dieting and intentional weight loss pursuits nearly always result in chaos, irregularity, and a loss of control around food. Of course, Diet Culture tells us we are to blame for this. It tells us if we just had more willpower, we could overcome our biology.

Developing a positive relationship with food leads to the sense of control around food we often look for through dieting. By addressing feelings of deprivation and shame, you can begin to develop healthier behaviors around food; in other words, foods that you used to experience intense cravings for will move into neutral territory. Practicing full permission to eat all foods opens them up to being enjoyed in an amount that feels both physically and mentally satisfying.

Many people in the early stages of this journey feel uncertain that they will ever achieve neutrality around the foods they have felt such a strong, intense pull toward for so long. Distrust in our bodies is powerful, and it is one of the major consequences of Diet Culture's influence. Your own personal experience with this process will be the antidote.

A key factor in breaking free from dieting is shifting away from a focus on weight and weight loss. In short, weight is not a reliable indicator of health (Bacon and Aphramor 2011; Bacon and Aphramor 2014). Although your weight may change when you engage in healthy behavior, not all weight changes are signs of good health. In the vast majority of cases, the behavior changes themselves are responsible for improvements in health (i.e., engaging in more joyful movement or engaging in less chaotic eating related to healing your relationship with food). Weight change is simply a common side effect of behavior changes along with shifts in health.

This is an important distinction because our bodies protect against intentional weight loss (Dulloo 2012). Therefore, weight loss is a very unlikely result of truly nourishing, supportive, healthy behavior changes. Many people will not lose weight in the long term when engaging in healthy behavior changes. And yet, their health will nonetheless improve. Ultimately, using weight as a measuring stick for health is misguided.

The relationship between weight and health is inaccurately portrayed in our culture (Bacon and Aphramor 2011). Many assumptions about weight and health are embedded deeply into the fabric of our society. Common assumptions include:

- Fat causes death.

- Fat causes disease.

- Weight loss prolongs life.

- Anyone can lose weight, if they try hard enough, by making adjustments in diet and exercise.

- The pursuit of weight loss is a positive goal.

- The only way someone in a larger body can improve their health is through intentional weight loss.

(Bacon and Aphramor 2011)

A growing body of research is challenging these long-held assumptions (Harrison 2019; Bacon and Aphramor 2014). And, in fact, a deeper look at much of the current weight science research shows fundamental flaws. For example, "long-term" weight loss success is defined as keeping the weight off for a year and a half, although most people will actually regain lost weight up to five years after a weight loss attempt. This finding ultimately skews the big picture of the sustainability of intentional weight loss pursuits.

Giving up a focus on weight can be challenging because our beliefs about the value of this measurement are deeply embedded in our culture, including our medical industry. Recommendations for weight loss at the doctor's office are commonplace, even when the

purpose of the visit has no relevance to weight
(i.e., an earache or the flu).

Here are some tips that will help you resist the urge
to focus on your weight:

- Stop weighing yourself at home.

- Listen to and honor your body's cues for how
  much to eat.

- Stop measuring success based on how your clothes
  fit or any other measure of the size of your body.

- Engage in healthy, supportive behavior changes
  rooted in addition rather than subtraction.

- Weigh biometric data (lab values, blood
  pressure, etc.).

- Consider your mental health.

UNDERSTANDING HOW DIETING SERVED YOU

Dieting has served a purpose in your life. It is important
to understand that purpose in order to find a new way
to meet an unmet need as you heal from dieting.

For many, dieting offers a powerful sense of control.
Controlling the minute details of what we consume can
make us feel as though we are in control of our bodies.
We believe that if we can control the number of calories
or the ratio of macronutrients we consume, we can control the size of our bodies and therefore the acceptance
we receive from others.

Alternatively, dieting can also provide us with a sense of control over our health. It can be scary to come to terms with the fragility of human existence. Controlling food intake, in an attempt to control health status, can feel safe and protective. And yet, ironically, doing so can be suffocating to the overall quality of our lives, essentially robbing us of the time we are trying to protect. In reality, diet and exercise comprise a very small percentage of the pie when considering all of the factors that impact health (such as socioeconomic status, gender, age, and genetics).

Dieting can also act as a distraction from more painful aspects of our lives. It is easier to avoid painful feelings when our brain space is being consumed by thoughts of calories, macronutrients, or whatever other variables a particular diet fixates on.

Finally, dieting can serve as a way to connect to others. Whether it's through shared experiences on the same diet, a weight loss support group, or mingling with coworkers over shared body dissatisfaction, dieting can fill a need for social connection. And, in this way, it can feel supportive and nurturing, despite the deep harm it causes.

So, dieting has served a purpose in your life. In order to leave dieting behind, you need to not only understand why it does not work, but also understand the needs it has met in your life. Doing so will allow you to meet those needs in more productive and supportive ways moving forward.

Counteracting the Effects of Social Media

One of the damaging impacts of Diet Culture is the obsession it creates around physical appearance. Women, in particular, have learned from a young age that their only valuable contribution is their appearance. They have also absorbed constant messaging that their bodies are wrong: Tone this, shrink that, wax this, and smooth that. The underlying message is that their bodies need to be fixed in order to compare to the societal ideal. The arbitrary societal ideal has become thin, white, able bodied, and cisgendered.

In modern day, social media fuels the already well established obsession around body appearance. Social media is home to the highlight reel in which individuals share the "best" (read: closest to the arbitrary societal ideal) images of themselves. This creates the illusion that other people's bodies always appear only at their very "best," rather than expressing the true natural diversity of women's bodies.

In essence, social media has become a battleground for comparison.

Although there are many ways social media can cause harm, there is also a lot of potential for its use as a tool for healing your relationships with food and body. There is a vibrant, active, engaged community of anti-diet and body acceptance activists who offer supportive, free content on their social media platforms.

Here are some tips for using social media to your advantage and minimizing the risk of becoming obsessed with body image. Please note: I use the word "fat" as a neutral descriptor in support of the fat acceptance movement.

1. **Unfollow or "mute" accounts that make you feel bad about yourself.** It is not unkind to mute the account of a friend who makes you question your worth every time you see their content. In fact, it may be much needed self-care on your journey.

2. **Follow accounts that show diverse bodies.** The vast majority of content we consume every day, voluntarily or not, shows one body type: the societal ideal. Of course you think your body is wrong when you are comparing it to one type of body out of the vast array of body types that exist. Start intentionally exposing yourself to other body types. Eliminate the accounts that repeatedly show bodies that are consistent with the societal ideal. Follow accounts of folks who are in marginalized bodies, including fat; Black, Indigenous, and People of Color; transgender; and disabled.

3. **Follow accounts that spread messages of body acceptance and food freedom.** Curate your feed to be a source of support to you on your journey. At some point, you may find the amount of positive messages around food and body to be overwhelming. It is okay to mute or unfollow some of these positive accounts at that point, as well. Allow your journey to progress and evolve.

4. **Connect with others on this journey through online or in-person support groups.** You will feel much better on this journey if you have people to connect with who relate to your experience.

Writing Exercise: Combating Body Shaming Messaging

Our culture is full of environments where people pick apart their own bodies and the bodies of others around them. Whether in the office, at a holiday party, with family, or on morning television talk shows, body shaming is all around us.

- When you hear body shaming messages, how might you begin to reframe them so they do not impact you in a negative way?

_____

_____

_____

_____

_____

- What content sources can you think of that portray and celebrate a diversity of body types, whether they are social media accounts, clothing brands, or anything else?

_____

_____

_____

_____

- Think about the people in your life. Who celebrates rather than shames body diversity?

_____

_____

_____

_____

_____

_____

_____

_____

_____

_____

_____

_____

_____

_____

_____

_____

_____

_____

Body Positivity and Health at Every Size

The appeals of dieting and pursuing weight loss are rooted in our belief that the appearance of our bodies is inherently wrong. Multiple systems benefit when we buy into this belief, including the diet industry and the patriarchy.

In the last 50 years, the body liberation movement has gained momentum. Originally born out of the fat acceptance movement, body liberation has invited us to look at our bodies in a new, more respectful way.

BODY POSITIVITY/BODY LIBERATION

Being Body Positive is . . . a way of living that gives you permission to love, care for, and take pleasure in your body throughout your lifespan.

—*Connie Sobczak, 2014*

Body positivity has roots in the fat acceptance movement. In 1967, Lew Louderback, a society-declared fat white male, wrote an article speaking out against size discrimination (Louderback 1967). In the article, he criticized the way "fat" people were treated in America and called out size discrimination in the workplace. Two years later, in 1969, the National Association to Advance Fat Acceptance was founded with a mission of eliminating discrimination based on body size.

Body positivity has expanded over the years to include the many ways our bodies are scrutinized by the wider culture. In 1996, The Body Positive was founded by Connie Sobczak and Elizabeth Scott. This organization had the mission of creating a community that would help people free themselves from the suffocating societal messages about bodies. This is where the term "body positivity" was born. Since gaining momentum over the past couple of decades, the term "body positivity" has shifted away from its original meaning in many contexts.

There are many criticisms of the way body positivity has evolved in recent years. One critique is that it continues to center on a person's body as a core piece of their identity. Shifting from a focus on body negativity to one on body positivity is certainly a step in the right direction, but that still supports a continued fixation on the body. Additionally, as body positivity has become more mainstream, it has focused on bodies that are still in many ways similar to the societal ideal, rather than those that are the most marginalized. In other words, the faces of body positivity have become *slightly less thin*, white, conventionally beautiful, cisgender, able-bodied women. True body positivity should center on the most marginalized bodies.

Body liberation is a newer concept that aims to intentionally steer clear of the mainstream and diluted "body positivity" message. Instead, it focuses on the goal of shifting away from trying to love the appearance of your body to finding a more neutral relationship to it.

In many ways, finding positive emotions toward our bodies can feel like an impossible task. When we shift to body neutrality, the task feels more accessible for many. The goal is not to love your body. The goal is for how you feel about the appearance of your body to not get in the way of how you live your life or how you take care of yourself. The goal is to lessen the impact of body thoughts on your daily life so that you can invest your time and energy into what is most important to you. Body liberation, like food freedom, is about reclaiming the life that our culture has stolen from you.

DIVERSITY AND INCLUSION

There has been a push for increased diversity of models in the fashion industry in recent years. While there is no doubt that a shift has occurred, there continue to be hiccups:

- Brands like Target, H&M, and Aerie need to hire models of more varied body sizes. Although some of these stores now have larger models in their advertising, their clothing sections in stores are not well managed. In some cases, the larger-sized clothing is only found on one rack within a store. This observation is especially disturbing, considering that two-thirds of Americans wear clothing in this category. ModCloth, an online-only retailer, has merged its straight-sized and "plus"-sized clothing lines to offer "extended sizing."

- In June 2019, an article in *The Telegraph* was released trashing Nike's decision to include plus-sized mannequins in its London store. The article suggested that the larger-sized mannequin could not possibly be "going for a run" and made erroneous claims about its presumed health status.

- In January 2020, Jillian Michaels, a former trainer on the popular television show *The Biggest Loser*, made a comment on *BuzzFeed News* criticizing the singer Lizzo's body. She asked, "Why should we celebrate her body? Because it's not going to be great if she gets diabetes."

There have certainly been steps in the right direction regarding weight inclusivity and representation in the media. However, there are equal and opposite reactions from a deeply fat-phobic culture. In short, there is still a long way to go.

HEALTH AT EVERY SIZE

The Health at Every Size movement aims to shift the focus of health away from body size manipulation and toward healthy behaviors and access to health resources for people of all sizes. In 2003, the Association for Size Diversity and Health (ASDAH) was formed and the Health at Every Size (HAES) model was born. This approach is comprised of five principles:

1. Weight Inclusivity: **Accept and respect the inherent diversity of body shapes and sizes, and reject the idealizing or pathologizing of specific weights.**

2. Health Enhancement: **Support health policies that improve and equalize access to information and services, and personal practices that improve human well-being, including attention to individual physical, economic, social, spiritual, emotional, and other needs.**

3. Respectful Care: **Acknowledge our biases, and work to end weight discrimination, weight stigma, and weight bias. Provide information and services from an understanding that socioeconomic status, race, gender, sexual orientation, age, and other identities impact weight stigma, and support environments that address these inequities.**

4. Eating for Well-Being: **Promote flexible, individualized eating based on hunger, satiety, nutritional needs, and pleasure, rather than any externally regulated eating plan focused on weight control.**

5. Life-Enhancing Movement: **Support physical activities that allow people of all sizes, abilities, and interests to engage in enjoyable movement to the degree that they choose.**

(Association for Size Diversity and Health 2020)

A common misconception about Health at Every Size is that it stands for "Healthy" at Every Size. This implies that people of all sizes are healthy or can be healthy at any size. It is true that people can be healthy at a much wider range of sizes than our culture suggests; however, this is not at the core of the movement. At the core of the movement is a push for an end to size-based discrimination and weight stigma, and support for health behaviors and health resources for people of all sizes, without a focus on purposeful body size manipulation.

There are many factors at play when considering individual health, including socioeconomic status, genetics, and the experience of oppression. However, our current weight-centric medical system distills health down to a focus on weight and weight loss. Rather than considering the impacts of the multifaceted variables at play, doctors and other health professionals prescribe weight loss and send patients on their way. The use of the Body Mass Index (BMI) to diagnose weight as a disease has become disconcertingly commonplace.

The BMI was created in the early 19th century by an astronomer in order to assess the weight of a small group of European participants at the population level. The equation was never meant to be used on the individual level, much less to diagnose disease risk. And it certainly does not account for variability in natural body types across different ethnicities, genders, or age groups. The categories (underweight, normal, overweight, and obese) are completely arbitrary and inherently stigmatizing by making assumptions about health status based on body size.

To say someone is "overweight" is to assume that there is one appropriate size for a body to be, rather than accounting for the vast diversity in body size that naturally exists. Furthermore, to say someone is "obese," which translates to "someone who has eaten themselves fat," shows there is inherent stereotyping about someone's behavior based on their body size. Perhaps most ironic of all, people in the "overweight" category have actually been shown to have the highest life expectancy (O'Hara and Taylor 2018; Waaler 1984).

A focus on weight in managing health is not only misguided, but also harmful. When you try to control your body weight by manipulating food intake and exercise, your body responds by driving you to regain lost weight. We have known for some time that purposeful manipulation of body size does not work. In fact, the National Institutes of Health reached this consensus in 1992 (Technology Assessment Conference Panel 1992). At the time, they concluded that intentional weight loss pursuits had a consistent pattern of resulting in weight regain within five years.

The reason for this near-perfect weight regain pattern is that our bodies actively respond to shifts in calorie intake and body weight in the same way they respond to shifts in body temperature. Imagine if you were playing basketball outside in 90-degree weather. Your body would start to produce sweat in an attempt to cool you down to the temperature that it feels comfortable and safe at. The same compensatory mechanisms occur to protect your body's setpoint weight (Bacon and Aph-ramor 2011). Setpoint weight is the weight range that your body is calibrated to protect at any particular time. An individual's setpoint weight will shift over their life as a result of medication, dieting, significant life events, aging, and hormonal shifts. It is important to note that a body protects weight that it has already gained more vigilantly than it protects against weight gain. In other words, it is far more likely that the setpoint will adjust in the upward direction over the lifespan rather than in the downward direction. Setpoint weight should not be confused with the societally constructed "normal weight" ranges, as, again, BMI is deeply flawed.

Many studies on the relationship between ill health and weight do not control for two very important factors: the experience of weight stigma and the presence of weight cycling (the repeated loss and regain of weight). Both of these factors have well established negative impacts on health.

Furthermore, internalized fat-phobia impacts behavior. For example, if a fat person internalizes the message that they are lazy and make unhealthy choices, their behaviors begin to reflect this belief about themselves (Chastain 2018). In this way, beliefs about oneself being unhealthy become a self-fulfilling prophecy.

Finally, science is inherently biased. It is impacted by the perceptions and widely held beliefs of the wider culture, which influence the questions that are asked.

Fat-phobia is embedded into the fabric of our culture and, therefore, into the research that is being conducted in this area.

Most important of all, regardless of the health status of a fat person, all people deserve respectful care that is not rooted in weight stigma or size discrimination.

The Health at Every Size model is a framework for an essential task: Fight weight stigma and discrimination in health care and promote health access and behaviors for people of all sizes. Individual work on fat acceptance, body liberation, and food freedom can absolutely be helpful, but it will not change the fact that we exist in a climate that treats fat people poorly.

Dieting causes harm by disconnecting us from our bodies. Rather than taking care of our bodies by meeting the needs they communicate to us, we prioritize the diet rules.

- In what ways have your feelings about the appearance of your body impacted how you have taken care of yourself?

_____

_____

_____

_____

_____

_____

_____

_____

_____

_____

_____

_____

Putting It Together

Diet Culture is the result of a dynamic interplay of deep cultural norms and beliefs. If we did not believe that our bodies were wrong, that being fat was inherently unhealthy and unattractive, that the appearance of our bodies was a key element of our worth, then diets would not be appealing. In order to heal our relationships with food and our bodies, we need to understand what is fueling the disorder: our culture. We need to unpack and challenge long-held beliefs about weight and health.

Let's check in with the exercises we have gone through so far:

- What do you ultimately hope to gain from this book?

- What is your vision for your relationship with food?

- What do you hope to gain more time for when you spend less time concerned about food and your body?

- Consider the factors that have contributed to your relationship with food today.

- What void has dieting filled in your life?

- Curate your social media accounts to serve your healing journey.

- What are some messages that you can tell yourself to counteract body-shaming environments?

- In what ways have your past feelings about the appearance of your body affected how you have taken care of yourself?

Chapter Three

Listening to Your Body

Your body has so much wisdom to share with you about how to best care for it. We are all born with an innate ability to connect and respond to various body needs, and, therefore, we each have a very useful guide for our own body's care. However, this feedback is often extinguished by Diet Culture. When we are disconnected, we turn outward for guidance on what, when, and how much to eat. Rather than tuning into what sounds good to our own bodies, we rely on rules and guidelines. Each choice we make based on something external to ourselves reaffirms this distrust in our own body. We continue to subscribe to the belief that our bodies could not possibly guide us around eating. We buy into the fear that if we listened to our bodies, all we would ever choose to eat would be French fries and cake. Ironically, the distrust we have in our bodies is what fuels the chaotic behavior around food that we fear. When we tune in to our bodies' cues, we find a level of trust we never knew we could foster.

When we are disconnected from our bodies' wisdom around food, we are also unlikely to have awareness around other needs. This state may lead to mindless emotional eating that blocks us from meeting the deeper emotional need beneath the surface. Although there is nothing morally wrong with emotional eating and it can absolutely serve many purposes, if used to dull painful emotions, it can prevent those emotions from being addressed more directly.

Your body also has a lot of wisdom to share regarding the stress you experience in your life. Some amount of stress is perfectly normal, but too much stress can begin to infect multiple facets of your life, ultimately impacting your health and well-being. In this chapter, we will discuss various ways in which your body provides you with feedback, including hunger, satisfaction, emotional eating, and stress. We will also cover how you can reconnect to the cues around these variables so you can better show up for your body's needs.

Feeling Hungry and Feeling Satisfied

Hunger and satisfaction are two of the most basic and supportive body cues we have. Without them, we would not be motivated to take in energy in the form of food. In short, we would not survive. Diet Culture makes hunger seem like an inconvenience, something to tame. In reality, our attempts to control hunger only serve to put us at war with our bodies. And biology always wins. Diet Culture makes satisfaction seem like a code to crack with the fewest calories possible. But hunger and satisfaction are actually very intuitive when we attempt to control them. When we embrace hunger and the satisfaction we experience with food, we start to find the peace we are looking for.

When we begin to understand the mechanics behind hunger and satisfaction, it becomes a lot easier to see why honoring and respecting these cues is so important on the journey to healing our relationships with food. Perhaps even more important on this journey is arriving at the understanding that you deserve to eat. You deserve to be satisfied, find pleasure, and be nourished by food.

Eating food is an essential function of being alive. Hunger is the vital biological cue that ensures we seek out food. In the same way we are motivated to cater to other basic needs like thirst and sleep, hunger signals ensure we are motivated to seek the energy needed to sustain life. In fact, the presence of hunger is a sign of good mental and physical health. During times of illness, hunger signals are often muted and do not return until the illness subsides.

Although Diet Culture may claim that hunger is something to be monitored and tamed, the truth is that hunger is a tool that supports us in meeting one of our most basic needs. Attempts to suppress hunger or keep it at bay ultimately backfire, causing that hunger to come back with double the intensity. But most important, when you try to suppress hunger, you are working in opposition to your body's needs. Doing so sends a clear message that there is a war between your mind and your body, a true disconnection.

Diet Culture also suggests that the amount of energy you need in a day is a definitive number and, thus, hunger cues should be the same every day. However, it is completely normal for hunger levels to fluctuate on a daily basis. This fluctuation is due, in part, to shifts in resting energy needs. Resting energy needs account for basic bodily functions like blood flow, food digestion, and brain functioning. These energy needs shift constantly for a variety of reasons.

Additionally, levels of physical movement throughout the day or week impact hunger levels. Extra movement you engaged in two days ago could impact your hunger levels today as your body continues to recover and rebuild from that expenditure. Other factors that contribute to fluctuating hunger levels include dieting, medication, illness, menstruation, and physical or emotional stress.

Dieting increases hunger levels immensely by causing the body to increase the production of hunger hormones in an attempt to return to its starting weight or, in many cases, reach a higher weight (Dulloo 2012).

There are also different types of hunger that meet different needs. Biological hunger results from the physical need for energy to survive. It is often characterized by physical cues like a headache or rumbling stomach. Our bodies need a consistent intake of energy to maintain basic bodily functions, as well as any additional physical expenditure.

Emotional hunger may result from events like wanting to share a celebratory birthday cake with a loved one. It also may result from a need for comfort. Food can satisfy a need for soothing. Emotional hunger and emotional eating are essentially the impacts of emotions on one's behavior around food.

Taste hunger results from a desire to experience a particular food in the absence of physical hunger—for example, when you eat a delicious and satisfying meal and still crave a piece of chocolate cake for dessert. There is nothing inherently wrong with this desire. Honoring these types of cravings can often be supportive of a healthy relationship with food. Taste hunger is often criticized in Diet Culture because it is not a physical need for food.

Many factors contribute to the way we experience hunger. In many ways, we have been taught to distrust and fear hunger cues. However, when we work in conjunction with our cues rather than fighting against them, we can find a more peaceful way of meeting one of our bodies' most basic needs.

GETTING THE MOST OUT OF MEALTIME

In order to get the most out of mealtime, it can be helpful to consider the elements that contribute to a satisfying meal. Satisfaction from a meal means feeling content with the food you have eaten, both physically and mentally. Physically, it is a comfortable level of fullness in which you are no longer hungry, but also not overly full. Mentally, it is the absence of feeling deprived. It is having your food desires met. It is essential to have both mental and physical elements to experience true satisfaction. You can physically consume enough energy and still feel deprived if you did not eat what you desired.

Satisfaction is a major contributing factor to our behavior around food. When we are satisfied, we are content. When we are not satisfied, we become fixated on what we feel deprived of. This is a natural, supportive response to the feeling that our bodies do not have enough.

Satisfaction levels are influenced by our environment, the type of food, how that food aligns with what sounds good, how present we are with the sensory experience of the meal, the amount of food we enjoy, and the nutritional components of the food.

Although often overlooked, satisfaction can have a meaningful impact on our behavior around food. For example, with some curiosity and attention, you may learn that when you have a small egg and cheese wrap for breakfast, it satisfies your need for what sounds good but does not keep you sustained for very long. Alternatively, you may find that when you have a bowl of oatmeal with fruit, you feel physically sustained throughout the morning; however, you are reaching for food an hour later because this breakfast did not satisfy your taste hunger. Using satisfaction as a guide when making food choices can significantly change the way you relate to and behave around food.

Many times when you are dieting, you may feel frustrated by cravings for certain foods because you feel like you should be satisfied from having eaten enough calories. However, in this case, mental satisfaction was not achieved. Mental dissatisfaction can lead to a lot of chaos in our relationships with food, and many of us blame ourselves for not having the "willpower" to overcome it. In reality, meeting mental satisfaction needs is a key component to a peaceful relationship with food.

Here are some tips for finding satisfaction at mealtimes:

- **Set an intention to begin eating at a place of moderate hunger more often.** Beginning to eat in a ravenous state naturally leads to eating to an uncomfortably full state. Bring awareness to what moderate hunger feels like for you. Identify barriers to honoring your hunger at that level.

- **When you are deciding what to eat, bring awareness to what sounds good to you at that moment.** Ask yourself what taste, texture, temperature, and aroma of food are appealing at that time.

- **Trust your body to guide you.** Commit to giving yourself unconditional permission to eat the foods that sound good to you.

- **Explore eating with less distraction.** Although it isn't always possible, being present with the sensory experience of eating is often far more satisfying than distracted eating. Experiment with what it feels like to put your phone aside for a meal or purposefully eat at the kitchen table. Do not feel as if you have to do this every time you eat a meal, but allow yourself to experiment with it.

- **Explore mindful eating.** Experiment with eating the first few bites of a meal while paying full attention to the sensory qualities the food offers.

The more satisfaction you experience from a meal, the more present you will be with your life outside of the food. Be mindful that this could be a reason that you have used food control measures in the past: to avoid being present in your life. Depending on what life situations are present, showing up can feel scary or unsafe. Be gentle with yourself if you feel resistant to this process of letting go of food fixation.

When you feel ready, follow the aforementioned tips for experiencing more satisfaction at your meals.

Thought Exercise: What Is Making Me Hungry?

Over the next 24 hours, get curious about the factors that contribute to your desire to eat. Notice the types of hunger and the different cues that are present.

- You may notice that when you are hungry you start to think about food more, contemplating what you might want to eat for lunch.

- You may find you have a slight headache or a rumbling in your stomach.

- You may notice that your desire to eat is the result of a social gathering or an attempt to soothe an emotional need.

- Give yourself permission to observe without judgment, remembering that each of the different types of hunger are valid and serve to offer some kind of information.

The Myths Around Food and Sugar Addictions

Many people in our culture experience the feeling of being addicted to food. Both physical and mental food deprivation contribute to chaotic, obsessive, and compulsive feelings around food. These deprivations can trigger intense cravings for and fixations on food that will last until the desire or need has been met. This feeling is evolutionarily beneficial; when our ancestors did not have food available, they were motivated to get food by this type of fixation. When they finally found food, they would be motivated to overcompensate by eating much more than they needed in order to stock up fuel reserves to protect against future famine. This process was beneficial at a time when food was scarce.

Feeling addicted to sugar also makes a lot of sense, biologically. When total energy intake is diminished, sugar is the first and most urgent nutrient our body seeks. Sugar is the primary fuel source for the brain and, therefore, is a top priority. When energy intake needs are met but carbohydrate intake is not, the drive for sugar will still be extremely high because your brain's need for this nutrient remains a top priority to be met.

Think of the obsessions around food and sugar in comparison to other basic life needs. If you were deprived of water, you would be obsessed with water. If you had to pee, you would be overtaken by thoughts of finding a bathroom. And if you were deprived of oxygen, you would feel a desperate need to breathe.

Because of your brain's reliance on sugar, when it is deprived in some way, you crave foods that contain sugar. Most of all, in these instances, you are driven to foods that offer high amounts of simple sugar. Think: white bread, candy, ice cream, cake, cookies, etc. It is not because those foods are inherently addictive. You are drawn to them because your brain has been deprived of sugar.

Many people worry that we live in an environment that constantly bombards us with advertisements for highly palatable foods. They worry that the constant messaging around food will drive us to eat more. In reality, as a culture, we are only susceptible to the messaging around food because of the epidemic of food deprivation we are in. Since, as a whole, we operate from a place of food scarcity (due to Diet Culture), we are highly vulnerable to messaging around food. When we eat intuitively and give ourselves full permission to eat all foods all the time, we are immune to the messaging around food because we are tuned in to our bodies' wants and needs. Again, it does not mean that we won't crave or enjoy those foods. However, we will not be coerced into wanting to eat large amounts of them after seeing an advertisement.

The feeling of food addiction is a very real experience. The urgent, obsessive, chaotic draw to certain foods is real. However, the way we approach healing this behavior shifts when we better understand the cause: deprivation. Rather than avoiding the food as you might if you looked at it through the lens of addiction, when you understand it as a response to deprivation, you can work to allow yourself full permission in order to stabilize your relationship with that food in time. The former approach will only fuel the fire of obsession, fixation, and chaos.

Emotional Eating and How It Affects You

Emotional eating can be described as the impact of emotions on eating behaviors. Emotional eating has a negative connotation in our culture because, in a culture obsessed with thinness, eating outside of a physical need is seen as greedy, unnecessary, and a behavior in need of "fixing."

The irony is that, in a culture that provides the perfect environment for fixation on food by pushing diet mentality, emotional eating is a very common phenomenon. Food is more comforting and soothing when we have experienced food deprivation, whether it is physical or mental in nature. In other words, food is a more effective coping skill for people who have felt deprived of food in some way.

Emotional eating is a natural human behavior. It has a negative connotation in Diet Culture because anything that is not absolutely necessary food consumption threatens the fantasy of the thin ideal. But emotional eating is not always a destructive behavior. It can absolutely be an appropriate and supportive coping skill for difficult emotions. It can serve as a distraction technique in much the same way as watching a movie or reading a book can offer a break from deeper emotions.

There are many forms that emotional eating can take. It might even present itself as the absence of eating due to the experience of overwhelming emotions. Or, it may involve eating for social connection or celebration, or out of joy.

When emotional eating becomes a primary source of comfort or coping, it may be a disservice. Since it is a distraction mechanism, eating does not allow you to directly address the emotions that are troubling you. If you notice that food becomes a way of escaping or chronically avoiding deeper emotions, it may be supportive to start introducing different coping skills.

If emotional eating has been your only coping skill for some time, it may be the only coping skill that feels effective. Allow yourself full permission to use emotional eating as a coping skill during the process of introducing and exploring new ones.

The goal is not to eradicate emotional eating, because, again, emotional eating is a natural human behavior that can be supportive. The goal is to add more tools to your toolbox so you will be better supported and your emotions will be more directly addressed.

RECOGNIZING EMOTIONAL EATING

The first step in learning to recognize eating for emotional needs is building awareness and attunement around your body's cues for hunger and satisfaction. When you are not attuned to hunger and satiety cues, your body attempts to persuade you to eat and make up for what it feels deprived of. The experience can be very emotionally charged.

Once you feel adequately attuned to hunger cues and are consistently honoring them, you can start to develop awareness around eating outside of the intent of meeting that need. When you find yourself reaching for food, get curious about the reasons behind your urge. Remember to remain nonjudgmental.

In a large majority of cases when people feel they are eating emotionally, they are also eating out of some degree of an unmet physical or mental need. An unmet physical need for food can feel extremely emotional. You may experience irritation, anxiety, or anger when you are overly hungry (that dreaded "hangry" feeling). Furthermore, an emotional trigger like feeling stressed after a long day of work may coincide with a physical need for food after not eating for many hours. You may feel inclined to blame the hunger solely on the stress you are experiencing; however, your urge to eat may be partially fueled by the facts that it has been a long time since you have eaten and your body has a physical need for energy.

Eating in the absence of hunger may also be a response to the body trying to overcompensate for not being adequately nourished earlier in the day. Once again, this act can feel very emotionally charged in the moment, especially when you feel guilt and shame for being driven to eat more food in the absence of physical hunger. Furthermore, often the foods we are drawn to at these times are ones that provide quick energy, like simple carbohydrates and high-fat foods. Sometimes clients I work with experience this feeling after dinner. They find themselves grazing as soon as they walk in the door from work. They eat a full dinner. And then, after dinner, they find themselves grazing more. They are sure their actions must be strictly emotional eating because they are not physically hungry anymore. However, this desire to keep eating can be a result of not eating enough earlier in the day, or a very normal reaction to taste hunger.

Working to honor hunger more consistently throughout the day addresses a certain degree of the chaos we experience while doing what we feel is emotional eating.

Here are a few indications that you might be eating to meet emotional rather than physical needs:

- You do not experience physical sensations of hunger (empty feeling in your stomach, grumbling stomach, headache, etc.).

- You have been experiencing intense emotions lately (anxiety, sadness, depression, etc.).

- You have been eating consistently and adequately throughout the day for a while.

- You feel sensations of fullness and satiety (stomach feels full and satisfied).

- When you tune in to ask yourself what you are feeling, you can identify an emotional need in this moment (feeling sad, angry, anxious, etc.).

The first step to understanding your own emotional eating habits is to develop awareness. The awareness will allow you to get a sense for what is driving the behavior. The second step is to channel self-compassion and understand that the goal is not to eliminate emotional eating. If you feel the goal is to eliminate emotional eating, then you set yourself up for feeling deprived. Furthermore, there is no need to eliminate emotional eating, because it is a natural part of life. A healthy relationship with food absolutely includes some degree of emotional eating.

Allow yourself full permission to eat emotionally, and commit to bringing awareness to the emotions you are experiencing underneath.

COPING WITH EMOTIONAL EATING

Once you develop awareness around eating for comfort and soothing, you can start to address the emotions that are underneath. Awareness is the first and most powerful step. Even if you make no changes to the way that you are eating in response to emotions, awareness gives you the power to address your emotions more directly. Doing so serves your overall mental and physical health, independent of food intake.

When you find yourself reaching for food, get curious about what is driving you to do so. Is it purely physical hunger? Do you not sense hunger at all? If that's the case, you can consider this desire for food as a red flag that something deeper might be going on. Ask yourself what emotion you are feeling. If doing so feels too difficult, check in with how your day is going. Check in with what situations you have encountered. How are you feeling physically? Tired, drained, or energized? This information may open you up to better understanding what emotions you are feeling. Sometimes, it can even be helpful to look at a list of emotions so you can have some to choose from and match to how you are feeling.

Once you identify the emotion you are feeling, ask yourself what you might need. If the emotion you are feeling is anxiety or stress, maybe what you need is to cancel some plans for the night. Maybe you need to call a friend to come over and talk. Maybe you just need to vent to someone over the phone. Maybe you need to journal or take a five-minute walk or do a ten-minute yoga video. The possibilities are endless and completely individualized. Once you are able to identify the emotion you are feeling, you will better understand what might serve you in that moment.

Do not stop yourself from using food for comfort if that is what your body is driving you toward in the moment.

As soon as you restrict yourself from turning to food, your body will sense mental deprivation. If turning to food to cope with emotions has been your primary coping skill, it is going to be the most effective skill in that moment. You do not need to take that away from yourself. And, ultimately, trying to stop yourself from using food for comfort will only fuel this behavior in the long run.

If you are reading this and thinking of all the ways emotional eating does not serve you and does not feel good, I understand. Still, the answer is not to purposefully restrict yourself from emotional eating all together.

Once you develop more coping skills for mindfully and directly addressing your emotions, emotional eating will take its rightful place as simply one gentle way of coping in addition to a toolbox full of other skills.

Thought Exercise: Coping Skill Exploration

Food can sometimes serve as a way to push away or soothe difficult emotions.

- Think about a time when you used food to cope.
- What were you feeling?
- What might have addressed that feeling more directly?

Remember that the goal is not to eliminate emotional eating, and remember that there is nothing wrong with this coping skill.

MANAGING STRESS

Stress is nearly impossible to avoid in our fast-paced culture. A need to cope with stress is a common reason to turn to food for comfort. Let's not forget that when we have been deprived of food in some way throughout our lives, food delivers a higher reward to our brain. In other words, food is more comforting to those who have dieted. Eating food is a more effective coping mechanism for dealing with stress or other emotions if you have experienced deprivation of food in the past.

However, eating food to cope with stress does not deal with the source of your mental discomfort. If the source is not addressed, the stress will continue to be an issue.

There are many ways to deal with stress in the short term. This may include breathing exercises, joyful movement, or simply reading a book to take your mind away from the stressful variable. But the most effective method for dealing with stress is taking stock of priorities and rearranging them in whatever way is realistic. If work is a major stressor and there is no expectation of things shifting for the better, it may be time to consider a new job. If a relationship is a primary stressor, it may be time to consider having difficult conversations or seeking help from a professional. Finding a professional therapist you trust to work with can be a game changer.

If stress is present in a significant way in your life, the most important thing you can do is find a way to directly alleviate that stress. Do not rip away your primary coping skill of emotional eating. Emotional eating may be uncomfortable, and it may not be serving you, but the most critical need is to find a way to manage the stress more directly. Then, as discussed above, as you work on developing other coping skills, emotional eating will take its rightful place as simply one of many skills that you use.

In short, if you are eating to cope with stress, you need to find a way to alleviate that stress directly.

Writing Exercise: Stress Relief

Think about a source of stress in your life right now.
It could be your job, a relationship, or something financial.

- Write about something you may be able to do to
alleviate some of this stress.

_____

_____

_____

_____

_____

_____

_____

- Can you set some boundaries in a particular relationship as you do your own healing?

_____

_____

_____

_____

_____

_____

_____

- Can you make a commitment to take your designated lunch break every day, rather than working through it?

_____

_____

_____

_____

_____

_____

_____

- The goal is to alleviate some of the stress caused by a particular factor in your life.

_____

_____

_____

_____

_____

_____

_____

_____

Mindful Eating

Mindful eating has roots in Buddhism and the practice of mindful meditation. In short, mindful eating is the act of being present with your meal. It is similar to Intuitive Eating in that it is a type of internally regulated eating (Satter 2020). Many applications of mindful eating have been spoiled by diet mentality. It has been viewed as a tool for eating less or, in other words, weight management. In reality, mindful eating is about enhancing the satisfaction, joy, and pleasure experienced in a meal. It has nothing to do with a goal of eating less or losing weight.

Practicing mindful eating involves bringing awareness to the sensory qualities of the food you are eating, as well as the environment in which you are having your meal. It may involve curating your environment so you have less distractions and can pay more attention to the food you are eating.

HOW TO REDUCE DISTRACTED EATING

Distracted eating is the act of eating while your attention is elsewhere. It can include watching Netflix, scrolling on your phone, eating quickly while preparing food for others, or eating on the go. When you are paying attention elsewhere while eating, it is challenging to connect to your body's cues, as well as to fully experience satisfaction and enjoyment from eating.

When you detach mentally from the eating process, you rob yourself of the mental satisfaction gained from enjoying food that your body is craving. Reducing distracted eating can support a healthy, more pleasurable relationship with food.

The goal is not to eliminate distracted eating, but rather to allow yourself to explore how your level of mental presence affects the amount of satisfaction you get out of a meal. Become curious about your satisfaction and pleasure when you eat a meal while watching a show compared to when you eat a meal while paying more attention to the sensations you are experiencing from the food.

This task, like all the content in this book, is not pass or fail, but rather an invitation to explore the feedback your body is giving you. This feedback will allow you to make decisions that are aligned with what serves you the best.

Distracted eating, particularly in our culture, is somewhat unavoidable. It will absolutely happen sometimes, and that is okay. There is nothing morally wrong with distracted eating. Again, Diet Culture demonizes any kind of eating that might lead to eating slightly more than is absolutely physically necessary. This is an unfounded fear that we do not need to continue to buy into.

If you get curious about distracted eating, rather than allowing yourself to get sucked into a shame spiral about it (feeling like a bad person because you eat mindlessly while watching Netflix), then you might become aware of the reasons behind why you are eating this way. This realization may be far more important than trying to blindly eliminate the behavior.

For example, maybe you are eating while scrolling on your phone or watching Netflix because you are dealing with a high amount of stress at work and this experience seems to soothe you. In this case, the answer is not to rip away the coping mechanism of eating while watching Netflix, but rather to address the chronic high level of stress you are experiencing. Recognize that you are worthy of having that stress dealt with; don't punish yourself for the resulting coping skills that surface.

Once you bring attention and awareness to the reason behind the distracted eating behavior, you will be better able to address that cause, and the distracted eating may naturally lessen.

Again, the goal is not to eliminate distracted eating. The goal is to become curious about why this behavior exists. Become curious about the feelings and judgments that come up regarding this behavior. If you feel guilt and shame around it, consider why that is. Is it because of the impact you fear it may have on your body if you eat a bit more than you physically need? Understanding the feelings you have about this behavior will help you heal it.

MINDFUL EATING AND INTUITIVE EATING

Mindful eating is distinct from Intuitive Eating. However, they both fall under the category of internally regulated eating practices. While Intuitive Eating was created by two Registered Dietitians in the mid-1990s, mindful eating has roots in Buddhism. Mindful eating is a practice that focuses on being present with the sensational experience of eating, as well as a connection to hunger and fullness. In this way, it overlaps with several Intuitive Eating principles, including honoring hunger, feeling fullness, and discovering satisfaction.

Intuitive Eating encourages an exploration of mindful eating within its framework. Being present with the sensory experience of eating is important for experiencing the satisfaction that is so important for a healthy relationship with food.

However, Intuitive Eating is a much more comprehensive approach in that it also encourages challenging cultural norms of Diet Culture with its principles of rejecting the diet mentality and challenging the food police. It also includes principles that address shifting your relationship to movement, coping with emotions with kindness, and respecting your body.

Intuitive Eating is a unique framework that aims to help people heal their relationship with food and body so they can be more present in their lives.

In sum, mindful eating is compatible with Intuitive Eating. However, they are each distinct ways of thinking about the reason for, and approach to, eating.

INTUITIVE EATING ON THE GO

Eating on the go in our culture is practically unavoidable. One of the simplest and most effective ways to practice Intuitive Eating on the go is to have snacks available. Whether you keep them in your car or at your desk, or make it a priority to remember to grab something before leaving the house, having food available for when hunger arises is a great way to support a healthy relationship with food. When you find yourself overly hungry or ravenous, it becomes challenging to meet your body's needs in a peaceful way. Keeping snacks available allows you to nourish your body in the way it deserves.

Commit to bringing awareness to various hunger cues throughout the day. Become familiar with the sensations of hunger you experience in your unique body. They may include an empty feeling in your stomach, a grumbling stomach, headache, thoughts about food, irritability, etc. Once you develop more of an awareness around what these cues feel like, you can commit to honoring your hunger more consistently throughout the day.

Another way to practice Intuitive Eating on the go is to intentionally consider in advance what foods usually sound good to you during the day. Consider your preferences. Rather than filling your glove compartment with random foods that you do not even enjoy, try to stock up on foods that usually do sound appealing to you. This list may take some time to figure out. Considering what foods are satisfying to you probably hasn't been a top priority in the past. But, discovering satisfaction is fundamental to the Intuitive Eating journey.

Another way to practice Intuitive Eating on the go is to bring awareness to the negative thoughts that come up around food or your body throughout the day. Once you build awareness around the types of thoughts that surface, you can begin to challenge them.

Intuitive Eating is not a one-size-fits-all approach. It is individualized and adaptable to each person's unique situation. There are many ways to incorporate the approach that will align with eating on the go.

Mindful Eating Exercise

This exercise can be practiced pretty much anywhere.

Choose a food that sounds good to you or that you have readily available. Ideally, choose a food that you are able to easily pick up with your fingers so you can get the full effect of all your senses being involved. However, if such a food is not available, you can still practice awareness around other sensations!

1. Even if your surroundings are full of distractions, bring your attention to the food in front of you. Take a few deep breaths to settle into the present moment.

2. Pick up the food, and start paying attention to the feel of it in your hands. Turn it over a few times, and think of a couple of adjectives to describe how it feels.

3. Bring the food to your nose and smell it. It may help to close your eyes for this part to get the full impact of the aroma.

4. Take a few moments to look at the food and take note of its appearance. Consider the color as well as texture.

5. Take a few deep breaths.

6. Take a small bite of the food, and allow it to rest in your mouth longer than you typically would.

7. Consider the flavor and the texture of the food.

8. Practice this exercise a few times with the same food.

9. After enjoying the food this way, take a moment to consider the overall satisfaction level of the experience. Consider how much you enjoyed the particular food.

You can practice this mindful eating exercise anywhere, anytime. Even if you can only get through a couple of the sensory awareness steps, it will be a powerful way of connecting to your body and bringing more satisfaction to your eating.

Putting It Together

In this chapter, we covered hunger and satisfaction in eating. We also discussed emotional eating in its various forms, and how to mindfully address emotions and stressors more directly. Finally, we covered mindful eating, and how to incorporate the approach in order to enhance satisfaction in eating.

Let's take a moment to reflect on the exercises that we have worked on so far:

- Contemplating your vision for your relationship with food

- Considering the factors that have contributed to your relationship with food today

- Thinking about the void dieting has filled in your life

- Curating your social media accounts to serve your healing journey

- Writing down how to counteract body-shaming environments

- Reflecting upon the ways in which your feelings about the appearance of your body have affected the way you have taken care of yourself

- Considering the factors that contribute to a desire to eat

- Exploring emotions that impact your desire to eat or not eat

- Writing down how to manage stressors in your life

- Practicing mindful eating

Take a moment to reexamine your responses to earlier exercises and consider if you have anything to add to them.

Chapter Four

Making Informed Choices

Somewhere along your journey to healing your rela-tionships with food and body, you will arrive at a place where you may be interested in making more inten-tional shifts around food in order to best serve yourself. When you do, allow yourself the time and permission to work on healing your relationships with food and body first. If you attempt to make these intentional shifts too early, you may unintentionally shift back into diet mentality and inflict the same damage on yourself that any other diet would.

Always come back to addition over subtraction. Examples of subtraction would be "healthy swaps," "cutting back," or "portion control" regarding particular foods. In contrast, gentle nutrition will consider the ways in which more nutritious foods, or sometimes just more food in general, can be incorporated to support your health and overall relationship with food.

Throughout this chapter, we will cover how to make food choices that honor both your body and mind. We will also cover practical skills like meal planning and grocery shopping. Finally, we will review how to incorporate new mood-boosting activities to enhance your overall quality of life. Remember that the goal is satisfaction, nourishment, and self-care. The goal is not to change the size or shape of your body. That is not how success is measured.

Nutrition and Nourishment

Honoring your health through gentle nutrition can serve your health both now and later. There is no need to sacrifice pleasure and satisfaction when being mindful of nutrition. And there is no reason to be restrictive to any degree. In fact, as we have discussed, any type of restriction will backfire. Rather than thinking of honoring your health through nutrition as something to perfect, think of it as a method of supporting your here-and-now body. Think of it as something to nourish and serve your body so you can be fully present for what is important to you in your life. And, again, use the concept of addition as a guide.

HONORING YOUR BODY WITH FOOD

In order to honor your body with food without getting sucked into the diet mentality, you have to set a few boundaries. First, avoid making food choices with the intent of trying to change the size or shape of your body. For example, seeking out lower-calorie foods is an example of making a choice with manipulating body size as the priority. In contrast, trust that your body will provide necessary feedback about the amounts and types of foods that you choose to eat, and will naturally self-regulate future choices to align with what serves it best.

Prioritize satisfaction and pleasure in eating. Trust that your body will lead you to a variety of different types of food when you give yourself full permission to eat all foods and various types are available. Many people are concerned that if they allow pleasure and satisfaction to guide their eating, they will only eat cookies and cake all day, every day. It is this distrust in our bodies that ends up sabotaging our behaviors. In reality, a strong pull toward foods like cookies and cake is often only a reaction to feelings of deprivation, guilt, and shame around those foods. If you ate cookies and cake all day for weeks on end, you would eventually reach a point where you crave something else instead. This outcome, of course, requires being attuned to what your body is asking for, as well as being adequately and consistently nourished.

It is hard to truly internalize this message until you experience it for yourself. Commit to exploring the concept of giving yourself full permission to eat the foods you have not trusted yourself around in the past.

In order to honor your body with food, you need to be aware of what foods are satisfying to you. That list of foods will change on a daily basis, so developing awareness and mindfulness around what your body is asking for is essential. Get in the habit of asking yourself before eating: What sounds good? Keep in mind that, if you are often in a ravenous state due to not eating consistently throughout the day, you will likely be drawn to high-calorie, high-fat, high-sugar foods in those moments. This desire is natural and protective. In these moments of depletion, your body wants the most quickly absorbed and most energy-dense nutrients to be available. There is nothing wrong with this feeling at all. But as you become more attuned to your body's needs and begin to honor its nourishment needs consistently throughout the day, you will find that the desperate need for these types of foods will subside. Of course, this easing does not mean you will never crave and want these foods; the cravings will just feel less urgent and chaotic.

Avoid any choices rooted in restriction or deprivation. The goal is not to eliminate, cut out, or cut back on any food. That way of thinking is diet mentality in its sneakiest form. The goal is to pay attention to what foods sound good to you and what foods feel good in your body. Doing so also means being mindful of any food intolerances. However, being mindful and aware of the fact that a particular food does not make you feel good does not automatically mean you can never enjoy that food. Continue to allow yourself full permission to eat the food with awareness. Give yourself the power of choosing how you would like to feel. Some days, you may decide the discomfort is worth the pleasure of enjoying the food. Other days, you may decide it is not. Both options are okay.

Remember the Intuitive Eating principle: Challenge the food police (Tribole and Resch 2012). Recognize if you have judgments around certain foods being good and others being bad. If you believe you really "shouldn't" have too much chocolate, this belief will negatively impact your behaviors around chocolate and contribute to a harmful relationship with that food.

In contrast, allow yourself full permission to eat the chocolate, while also being mindful and aware of how you feel when you eat it. Pay attention to which types and what amounts of that food are the most satisfying and pleasurable. Avoid creating a rule around how much is okay or good to have. Rules create a sense of scarcity and deprivation.

Make food choices that are aligned with your internal experience, rather than ones that are aligned with external rules. Instead of adding a protein to breakfast because someone told you that you should, consider adding it to breakfast because it sounds good or because you are exploring ways to feel more satisfied longer into the morning.

If you are someone who has never enjoyed nutrient-dense foods like whole grains, fruits, and vegetables, release yourself from any shame you may feel around this aversion. There could be various reasons for it. One may be the fact that you have always associated these foods with a diet or "being good" and other foods with being rebellious or "being bad." Another possible reason may be that you have not been exposed to them very much.

If doing so feels supportive to you at this point in your journey, consider experimenting with adding some of these foods to your day. Start small. Try adding a fruit for a snack or at breakfast. You could pick a vegetable to try roasting with dinner, or experiment with adding a salad with various vegetables.

Honoring your body with food can take many forms. To ensure this practice is not being conducted through the diet mentality lens, prioritize nutritious additions rather than subtractions.

MEAL PLANNING AND GROCERY SHOPPING

Diet Culture does not own meal planning and grocery shopping. These practices can be extremely supportive of self-care, completely separate from the intention of manipulating body size.

For many people, meal planning can remind them of being "on the wagon" when dieting. In much the same way that many people have closely associated exercise with dieting, meal planning can feel like something you want to rebel against. It can especially feel like this if there is rigidity in the meal plan and a sense of shame for not following it.

However, you can begin to shift the way you think about meal planning when you release a restricted calorie goal, allow it to be flexible, and intentionally choose to incorporate satisfying foods you love. If you always find yourself looking for something sweet after your meals, intentionally plan for this craving, and make a sweet food available at that time.

Meal planning when you are dieting is rigid and structured; however, meal planning with Intuitive Eating is flexible and meant to gently support you in meeting nourishment and satisfaction needs. If plans change one day, or you decide you don't have the energy to make the dinner you planned, allow for adaptation in the moment. If you decide what you planned to eat does not sound satisfying when the time comes to eat it, allow yourself the freedom to make another choice if that is financially and physically feasible at the time.

Along with meal planning, grocery shopping will set you up for meeting your body's nourishment needs throughout the week. However, grocery shopping can be a stressful experience, especially as you begin to experiment with full permission to eat all foods. It can feel overwhelming. Make a list ahead of time to ease some of the anxiety associated with grocery shopping. Remember that this list is also intended to be flexible. If you find something at the store that is not on your list but sounds amazing, you should absolutely allow yourself full permission to get that food as well, as long as doing so feels financially feasible for you.

As you make your grocery list, challenge yourself to add some of your fear foods. Fear foods can include foods you enjoyed as a kid, foods you feel you do not trust yourself around, or foods that you experience guilt or shame around when eating. Start to include these items on your grocery list. In time, and by giving yourself full permission, these foods will lose their power and emotional significance. In order to feel more comfortable with this challenge, try adding just one of these items to your list each time you go to the grocery store. Keep in mind that it is normal to find yourself eating a lot of these foods when you initially reintroduce them with full permission. As you learn to trust your body, your behavior around these foods will stabilize to more comfortable and supportive reactions.

Finally, make sure to plan for enough meals and snacks throughout the day and week. One of the most important aspects of Intuitive Eating is consistent and adequate nourishment. When you plan ahead, it makes these goals much more attainable.

Balanced Eating

Balanced eating is a natural outcome of the process of healing your relationship with food. Being in diet mentality may result in chaotic eating, oscillating between not eating enough and eating an uncomfortable amount. In contrast, Intuitive Eating results in equilibrium around foods that have long been feared, ultimately leading to regular portion sizes that feel comfortable and satisfying.

When balanced eating is seen as a tool for healing your relationship with food, rather than a natural outcome of it, balanced eating can very easily become a list of rules to follow. In other words, balanced eating can become a diet. Balanced eating should not be seen as a method or tool for achieving a healthy relationship with food, but rather as an outcome of this healing process. Allow it to unfold naturally in time.

Balanced eating can include eating consistently throughout the day in order to maintain nourishment levels, having a variety of satisfying nutrient-dense foods, and having a variety of satisfying play foods. Balanced eating may also include experimenting with incorporating a variety of different types of nutrients in meals and snacks in order to stay satiated for a comfortable period of time between meals.

Balanced eating is individualized and flexible. When you are tuned in to your body's needs, you might find that eating only eggs for breakfast does not sustain you as well as having eggs with toast and fruit does. A balanced and varied meal is often more satisfying. But, if you consider this philosophy through the lens of what you "should" eat, it can very easily be turned into a way of using external rules to guide your eating, rather than using your internal experience. Furthermore, some days, having a varied meal will not be achievable, and that is okay, too.

Part of balanced eating is understanding that sometimes meals and snacks will not be balanced. Sometimes a whole week of eating will not be balanced because life happens. This outcome is not a failure because balanced eating is not a diet. You are allowed to be human. You are allowed to prioritize other parts of your life when they demand it. And, if you are attuned to your body, when the dust settles you will be able to return to that connection and continue to support your body in a way that feels best for it most of the time.

Remember to return to a mind-set of addition rather than a mind-set of subtraction. Instead of assuming balanced eating must come from removing items from your plate, always consider what can be added instead.

Intuitive Meal Planning Exercise

Take a few minutes to consider options that sound good to you in each of the following categories:

- Breakfast
- Lunch
- Dinner
- Daytime snacks
- Nighttime snacks
- Beverages

1. Consider what you usually find yourself craving at each of these times. If doing so is difficult for you, take a few days to bring awareness to what sounds good to you right before eating at each of these times.

2. Consider the taste, temperature, and texture of foods that sound appealing.

3. Write a list of foods for each category listed above, and then use those lists to create a master list of your preferred or favorite foods.

4. Make sure you have several options for each category. (You might even explore recipes online or on Pinterest to get more ideas.)

Once you have this master list, plan out meals for the week ahead.

1. Make a list running from Sunday to Saturday (or whatever timeframe works most conveniently for your routine).

2. Plan out each meal and snack, allowing for flexibility, especially with snacks.

3. Make sure to consider ease of preparation, and make sure the list aligns with what is realistic for your routine.

4. Remember that this list is not a rigid plan. If you find that you are not in the mood for a particular meal that you planned on, you can always shift and make adjustments. However, having this master plan will ease a bit of your stress throughout the week.

Remember that there is absolutely nothing wrong with adding convenience foods to your master list. In fact, it is important that you include them. Having frozen or packaged meals and snacks available for busy days can be extremely supportive. If this meal plan is going to serve you, it must accommodate your needs. It needs to be reasonable and realistic. You can always add extra nutritional value, if you feel inclined to.

Boost Your Mood

Engaging in new activities can be a great way to practice self-care and boost your mood. Joyful movement is one type of activity that can support both physical and mental health.

It is important to shed any layers of guilt and shame regarding movement before you begin. Through the Diet Culture lens, not engaging in movement can feel shameful. The resulting feelings of guilt and shame become a barrier to exploring movement. Many people associate physical movement with weight loss attempts and thus with failure. It is important to dissociate movement from the intention of trying to change your body, so you can be more able to consider what type of movement will serve you physically, mentally, and spiritually.

You have likely heard that movement can contribute to improved mental health. It can relieve stress and provide much needed self-care. Commit to considering your personal experience with each type of movement, rather than considering what someone else does or what you think you should be engaging in.

Some types of movement may simply not be accessible for people with certain disabilities. Shifting the focus away from what others consider to be exercise and toward what feels like joyful movement for ourselves, in our own bodies in this particular period of our lives, will be helpful.

Rather than trying to engage in a movement activity that was externally suggested, invite yourself to choose a movement that sounds fun, enjoyable, and reasonable to you.

Engaging in movement is one way to support and foster a healthier relationship to your body. When you are choosing movement that serves you mentally, physically, and spiritually, you are connecting with your body. This choice opens you up to experiencing your body in new ways and developing a healthier relationship to it.

TRYING NEW THINGS

Healing your relationships with food and your body frees up a lot of time and energy. This new freedom can be both liberating and unsettling. Being fixated on food and your body may have been a mechanism you used to avoid being present in your life. It may have given you a purpose when you felt you did not have one. During this healing process, you will find a lot more space for new activities. Take advantage of this opportunity to seize your life back from Diet Culture.

Make a list of activities that you enjoy engaging in or that you have enjoyed in the past. It may also be helpful to make a list of activities that you have engaged in that you did not enjoy. The activities on your list do not have to be movement, per se. However, try to consider activities that will connect you to your body.

Some examples of activities that may connect you to your body include:

- Sitting outside in the sunshine and drawing or coloring

- Going bird-watching

- Yoga (inside or outside)

- Chair yoga

- Guided movement meditation

- Following a dance video

- Playing basketball with a friend

- Going for a walk

- Cooking

- Baking

- Listening to music

Whatever activity you choose should serve you and your body, as it is today. Become very curious about the intention behind your choice. Are you choosing the activity because you believe it is what you *should* choose?

- Are you choosing it because it is nostalgic and sounds enjoyable?

- Are you choosing it because it sounds new or exciting?

- Are you choosing it from a place of fear or shame?

Take note of the intention, and, if needed, adjust your list to best serve you. With time and exploration of different activities, you will ideally find some that you feel compelled to continue to engage in. If doing so feels important to you, prioritize carving out time for this activity in your week or month. Rather than framing this challenge as a pass-or-fail goal, try to frame it as a commitment to prioritizing yourself and your body's needs.

CONNECTING TO YOUR BODY

Fostering a connection between mind and body is a key step toward feeling better in your body. When you shift away from a focus on the appearance of your body and instead focus on what it feels like to exist in your body, you will start to see shifts in how you feel overall.

This growth is so important, because Diet Culture often brainwashes us into a hyperfocus on controlling food intake in an attempt to control the appearance of our bodies. This mentality ultimately leads to our identity becoming completely absorbed in the appearance of our bodies. How could it not, when all of our energy is being poured into creating or maintaining an image? Exploring and engaging in new activities in our lives will help us move away from putting all of our energy into manipulating the appearance of our bodies.

Even more, you deserve a life full of activities that serve your body and mind holistically. You deserve a life that feels connected and fulfilling.

As you explore these new types of activities, encourage yourself to be mindful of how they make you feel. If you experience joy, practice awareness. If you experience frustration, practice compassion and curiosity. Whatever you experience, be present for it.

Mood-Boosting Exercise

Commit to intentionally trying new activities on a regular basis. Choose a frequency that feels realistic for you right now (once per week, once per month, etc.). This activity could be something you have been interested in for a long time or something you used to enjoy that you want to get back into. It could also be a brand-new activity that you never considered trying.

Some ideas include:

- Playing an instrument
- Horseback riding
- Tai chi
- Yoga
- Going for a walk
- Going to a park with your dog
- Dancing to a dance video you find on YouTube

1. After you try a new activity, spend some time journaling about the experience. There is no right or wrong way to reflect on it. You may have loved the activity, you may have hated it, or you may feel somewhat indifferent.

2. Reflect on it and then decide which activities you would enjoy incorporating into your life in some way.

3. Keep a list of the activities you really enjoyed so you can pull from it the next time you want to have some fun.

Putting It Together

In this chapter, we discussed different ways to make choices around food that are supportive of your physical and mental health. We reviewed how to honor your body with food in a gentle way, as well as how to meal plan and grocery shop using Intuitive Eating as a guide.

We reviewed balanced eating and some of the misconceptions around it. And we discussed ways to boost your mood through engaging in activities that serve your unique body and mind.

Let's take a moment to reflect on exercises that we have worked on so far.

- Contemplating your vision for your relationship with food

- Considering the factors that have contributed to your relationship with food today

- Thinking about the void dieting has filled in your life

- Curating your social media accounts to serve your healing journey

- Writing down how to counteract body-shaming environments

- Reflecting upon the ways in which your feelings about the appearance of your body have affected the way you have taken care of yourself

- Considering the factors that contribute to a desire to eat

- Exploring emotions that impact your desire to eat or not eat

- Writing down how to manage stressors in your life

- Practicing mindful eating

- Planning out meals and grocery shopping

- Engaging in a mood-boosting activity

Take a moment to sit with earlier exercises, and consider if you have anything to add to them.

Chapter Five

You've Got This

One of the most common concerns while practicing Intuitive Eating is feeling stuck when it comes to actually applying the principles. Furthermore, trying to understand how to measure progress without the diet mentality lens can be confusing. Part of the issue is that healing your relationship with food is a nonlinear process with multiple twists and turns. Unlike dieting, there is no definitive Intuitive Eating rule book that dictates what you can eat and when. The wisdom of your own unique body, which you've likely been disconnected from for some time, becomes your guide. Furthermore, even once you begin to reconnect with your body and recognize cues, there is a deep sense of distrust in your body to work through.

Despite the somewhat precarious nature of this journey, there is structure that you can absolutely find, as long as you allow for some flexibility within it. Remember to reevaluate your goals throughout your journey to make sure they continue to support your current needs. At different points in your life, it is inevitable that your needs will shift.

In this chapter, we will review gentle, supportive goal-setting techniques. We will discuss how to set goals that align with your values in a way that will encourage you to achieve them. Furthermore, we will deconstruct what it means to make Intuitive Eating–aligned goals. You will also learn how to set a vision for your healing process moving forward.

It is important as you move forward that you commit to a journey that is driven by your own circumstances, values, and desires.

Setting Goals

Goal-setting around food and movement can be extremely supportive if done in a way that serves you. Goal-setting can also be suffocating if the goals are rooted in diet mentality. In that case, it can be destructive and will only lead to feelings of failure and hopelessness. In this section, you will be guided through setting goals that align with your own personal values and internal experiences.

Use the knowledge you have gained from this book to set goals that will support your journey to healing your relationships with food and body, as well as honoring your holistic health.

START SMART

SMART goals are an approach to effective goal-setting. The acronym "SMART" stands for Specific, Measurable, Achievable, Relevant, and Time-Based (Indeed.com 2020). When goals are set in a manner that is vague and nonspecific, it can be easy to lose sight and not follow through on them. However, when you create a vision for your goals, you will find clarity in the path to achieving them. This approach can help you set goals that allow you to create a vision around what will best support you on your life journey. Think of the process of setting SMART goals as an opportunity to explore your curiosities regarding what you need and what you want. Remember that goals aligned with the Intuitive

Eating approach are nonrestrictive. This means that rather than "cutting out" or "limiting" foods, you should concentrate your focus on adding satisfying, nutritionally diverse foods, as well as pleasurable activities, that will contribute to an overall improved quality of life.

Let's look at each element of a SMART goal:

Specific. Be specific when defining your goal. Create a vision in order to illuminate a path forward in achieving it. For example, a goal to start going to a dance class would be more specific than a goal to start engaging in joyful movement. Get clear on what you would like to do.

Measurable. Set goals that are quantifiable. Keep this part of the goal-setting process aligned with the Intuitive Eating approach by remembering that it is simply a vision. It is not a rule or something that can be passed or failed. It is simply meant to guide you. An example would be "Incorporating a satisfying vegetable into my breakfast two days per week." Take note of the "incorporating *into*" part; you are not cutting back or eliminating anything. Having a number of days per week to aim for allows this goal to be measurable.

Achievable. Consider what will be achievable and realistic, and what will best support your physical *and* mental health with consideration for your current life circumstances. Keep in mind what will feel best in your unique body. Setting an achievable goal is aligned with the Intuitive Eating approach because it encourages you to consider what serves you. Rather than aligning with what someone else says you should do, set an achievable goal that reflects what you can reasonably do. Again, consider not only what is physically feasible, but also what is mentally feasible. For example, if you have the goal of spending more time outdoors, yet you have a very hectic schedule, commit to spending some time outdoors once a month or once a week, whatever seems doable within the constraints of your schedule.

Relevant. Make sure that your goals are aligned with where you hope to be in your relationships with food and your body down the line. Consider the big picture. For example, setting a goal to go walking twice per week, even though you hate walking, would not be aligned with a goal of pursuing joyful movement that is both physically and mentally supportive.

Time-Based. Set a timeframe for when you will aim to achieve your goal. An example of this is planning to write a grocery list full of satisfying foods by Saturday evening, since you typically go grocery shopping on Sunday. Being specific with the timeframe allows for a concrete deadline that helps you prioritize and make space for certain tasks that are important to you.

SMART goals can help you develop a vision of where you hope to get to and build a roadmap to that destination. Setting goals can feel a bit triggering, particularly if you have come from diet after diet with rigid, structured rules around food and movement. There is often confusion around whether goal-setting can be aligned with the Intuitive Eating approach. This is because goal-setting in Diet Culture is so often so inextricably linked to changing the size or shape of our bodies that it feels tricky to unlink. Furthermore, the beginning stages of the Intuitive Eating journey focus on healing your relationships with food and body. As you progress through that healing process, eventually you will arrive at a place where supportive goal-setting around food and movement is appropriate and comfortable.

It is important to remind yourself that the goals you set are not pass or fail. Every obstacle is a learning opportunity and a chance to better understand yourself and your body. For instance, if you end up forgetting to write the grocery list before arriving at the store, allow yourself to be curious in a nonjudgmental way about why you forgot to write the list.

- Did you feel suffocated by the idea of writing a list?

- Did you simply not have the time?

- Did it not feel important to you?

All of these questions will provide valuable information as you move forward on your journey toward setting more aligned, achievable goals in the future. Having this awareness, compassion, and curiosity is meaningful progress all on its own.

Consider one of the goals you set for yourself when you first started reading this book. Develop a SMART goal approach for achieving the identified goal.

An example may look like the following:

Goal: I want to make healthier choices for my body that are not rooted in diet mentality. This first goal is my overall vision. It is a general goal that reflects where I would like to progress in my relationships with food and my body.

Now, let's refine that general goal to create a SMART goal:

Specific: I want to incorporate more satisfying vegetables in my meals.

Measurable: I will have one vegetable that sounds good to me at dinner twice per week.

Achievable: For the purposes of this example, let's assume I currently only very sporadically have a vegetable at dinner. It is not a consistent part of my routine right now. Let's assume I'm eating out for meals very often. This goal of having a vegetable at dinner twice per week seems achievable and appropriate given this fact, and I have considered the time, cost, and preparation that adding these vegetables will require.

Relevant: Since my overall goal is to make healthier choices for my body that are not rooted in diet mentality (external rules and guidelines), my goal feels aligned. I will make sure to choose vegetables that both sound good to me and feel good in my body to reinforce my connection to the feedback from my own body. Also, this goal sounds good to me in my own body and is not being driven by an external source or a belief that I "should" eat in this way.

Time-Based: I will incorporate one vegetable twice per week in my dinner by the end of this upcoming week. This adds a time-sensitive element to my goal.

ACHIEVING GOALS (AND GIVING YOURSELF A BREAK)

As we have discussed throughout this book, a powerful change to make when setting goals around food and movement is to shift to a perspective of addition rather than subtraction. Goals based around cutting out or limiting certain foods trigger the part of our brain that is rebellious and ultimately sets us up to have a chaotic relationship with food. Regardless of whether our intention for setting the limitation is based on a medical diagnosis or a desire to change the appearance of our body, our mind responds to the restrictions in the same way. Setting goals that are rooted in a mind-set of addition will be the most supportive method of achieving long-term behavior change.

Furthermore, shift away from a focus on intentional weight loss toward a focus on supportive healthy behaviors that are aligned with your personal values. Behavior-based goals are within your direct control.

In contrast, weight-based goals often clash with your biology and leave you feeling frustrated and discouraged. Furthermore, intentional weight loss is simply not necessary for improving and supporting health (Bacon and Aphramor 2014). Weight may naturally shift with behavior changes; however, it is not necessary to monitor or directly manipulate this variable, despite what our culture suggests. And, as we have discussed, attempts to control weight often backfire and result in worsened health outcomes (Bacon and Aphramor 2014).

It is also important to shift away from the pass/fail perspective that Diet Culture has instilled in your brain. If you feel like there is a "wagon" to be on, there will always be a wagon to fall off of when life happens. This outcome is not a failing on your own part, but rather a natural result of being human. Instead of considering situations that do not feel intuitive, aligned, or supportive as "falling off track," consider them opportunities for growth, understanding, and practicing self-compassion. Every situation is an opportunity to learn and can contribute to healing if approached in a nonjudgmental way.

Achieving goals in Diet Culture is generally measured by external, disconnected sources. Examples include weight loss, inches lost, progress photos, calories, macronutrients, steps walked, or generally "sticking to the plan." Move away from these external sources of measuring success in favor of a more internal process.

Allow yourself to measure progress by how you feel physically, mentally, and spiritually. Progress might feel like finding a renewed sense of peace around a previously feared food. You may find that although you used to be afraid to keep the food in the house because you would always find yourself eating past fullness, now you can have it in the house and feel very peaceful around it. You might choose to enjoy some at times and pass it up at other times because it doesn't sound good.

Progress might also feel like a renewed sense of energy as you learn to nourish yourself consistently throughout the day in a way that best supports your body. It may look like finding compassion and awareness in a moment of mindless eating, rather than getting lost in a spiral of guilt and shame. Or, your progress might feel stronger during a joyful movement exercise.

Redefine what progress looks like for you. Allow progress to be about feeling better in your body. Although you can absolutely set goals that are aligned with health and healing, allow your progress to be defined by how you feel, rather than by checking off the box of completing the task. And, of course, allow space for not always making choices aligned with your goal. Think of those nonaligned choices as expected parts of your journey and process, rather than shortcomings or signs of failure.

Shifting Measures of Success Exercise

Goals around food and body in Diet Culture are often rooted in external sources of measurement, such as calories eaten, food groups avoided, pounds lost, inches lost, number of steps walked, or minutes spent working out. Rather than being rooted in our own experiences and the sensations we have in our bodies, those goals are rooted in variables that disconnect us from our bodies.

- Make a list of the methods you have used in the past to measure success around food and body.

- How might you reframe your understanding of achievement to align with what you physically and mentally experience?

Continuing Your Practice

Once you open your eyes to the harms of Diet Culture, it is impossible to unsee them. You start recognizing them everywhere. Despite that, in many ways, Diet Culture messages are so deeply ingrained that they will continue to surface to the level of your awareness even after you have done a lot of healing work. This journey is deeply challenging, due to its countercultural nature. It goes against not only what we have experienced and grown up learning, but also much of the ideology and messaging we encounter daily in our lives. It is important to find ways to approach negative thoughts that will surface along the way on this journey. It is also important to find ways to enlist support on your journey, whether from people physically close to you in your life or others who are doing this work in places far away.

CHALLENGING NEGATIVE THOUGHTS

Negative thought patterns around food and body are the norms in our culture. We internalize negative messages, and they become part of our internal stories. During your healing journey, it will be crucial to develop awareness around these negative thought patterns. Some of these thoughts may be so deeply ingrained that it is difficult to recognize them as harmful. As you continue to peel back layers of awareness throughout this journey, you will uncover more long-held beliefs about food and body. In some cases, it may be worth challenging these thoughts and reframing them. In others, it will be important to simply allow space for these thoughts to exist and for the feelings that come along with them to surface. There is healing in feeling.

There are many types of negative thoughts that can present themselves when you consider the topics of food and body. Many can be linked back to messages from Diet Culture. Here are some examples of negative thoughts and ways to reframe them:

What if I gain weight on my journey to healing my relationship with food?

Reframe: I am experiencing fear around my body changing in a way that our culture tells me is inherently bad or wrong. It makes sense that I am having this fear, and I will allow myself to feel this fear. Also, I deserve the peaceful, healthy relationship with food that this process will give me. In time, my body will stabilize at a size that feels safe for it. I have the strength to adapt to making peace with my body.

My body looks terrible. I feel so fat.

Reframe: My body today does not look significantly different than it did yesterday, despite the massive shift in my thoughts about it today. The anxiety I'm experiencing around the appearance of my body today is likely linked to deeper anxieties I'm experiencing in my life. Furthermore, fat is not a feeling. Can I further unpack what I'm feeling? Am I feeling undesirable? Uncomfortable in my body? Sad? Mad? Also, "fat" is not a bad word. I will not continue to subscribe to the belief that it is bad to be fat.

What if I always eat in this uncontrollable way? What if the chaos doesn't stop? What if I can't really trust my body?

Reframe: The chaos I am feeling around food right now is a reaction to the physical and mental deprivation I have experienced previously. With time and by giving myself full permission to eat, I will find a place of balance and neutrality that is not only sustainable, but also comfortable and satisfying.

I'm so lazy.

Reframe: I am allowed to rest. It is supportive and healthy to allow myself rest. The most important act of self-care I can engage in today is to allow myself the rest I need. I am not lazy. When I am nourished and well rested, I will feel energized to engage in supportive movement.

Taking time to reframe negative thoughts is important as you learn to engage with food and your body in a new, more supportive way. There are so many harmful messages in our culture that will continue to trigger old patterns of thinking. The more time you spend practicing reframing negative thoughts, the more naturally it will come to you.

It is also important to mention that some negative thought patterns may be rooted in internalized fat-phobia or internalized weight stigma. These terms describe assumptions one makes about their own behaviors and characteristics that are the result of fat-phobic beliefs and the stigma around being in a particular-size body in our culture. It is impossible not to have some levels of internalized fat-phobia and weight stigma when we exist in a culture that passes them along to us. Even with deep work and healing around these beliefs, some amount will continue to exist within us. The goal is to minimize the amount that exists within us and the impact it has on our own self-care, as well as the impact it has on those around us.

An example of a negative thought rooted in internalized fat-phobia is when someone believes they are lazy. This belief may be tied to the wider perception that people who have larger bodies are lazy. When someone believes in their own laziness, that belief has an impact on the choices they make to take care of themselves. If one believes they are lazy, they are more likely to allow that belief to manifest in their life.

Keep in mind that although challenging negative thoughts is useful and necessary, it is also essential at times to simply allow space for feeling what you feel. You do not need to try to change your feelings. You do not need to mute your emotions. Even if your feelings are the result of a thought that is not rooted in truth, your feelings are still valid and need to be felt. Allowing space for your emotions essentially means bringing them to the surface and bringing much needed awareness to them.

REACHING OUT FOR SUPPORT

Support on your continued journey to healing your relationship with food and honoring your health and well-being is key to sticking with the process. Particularly, as you continue to expose the harmful food beliefs you have internalized, it can be unsettling to see all the areas of your life where these beliefs show up. They may show up in conversations with coworkers, at the gym, at your doctor's office, during family gatherings, in advertisements on the radio, and so on. It quickly becomes overwhelming and unavoidable.

Get connected to a group of people who understand the importance of healing your relationships with food and body. If you can find these people in person, that is helpful. But if you can't, there is a vibrant and active community online of anti-diet professionals, as well as many support groups on Facebook filled with folks going through this journey themselves. It can be so helpful to share your struggles and connect with those who understand them and are currently in the same place.

It will also be important, as you continue on your journey, to set boundaries around diet talk with friends and family members who are immersed in the dominant harmful beliefs around food and body. Furthermore, it might be helpful to introduce the people closest to you in your life to the concepts of Intuitive Eating so they can best support you on your journey. Doing so may very well impact their relationships with food and their bodies for the better, as well.

Finally, for more individualized support, it can be invaluable to work with a Certified Intuitive Eating Counselor or an Intuitive Eating–aligned dietitian or therapist on your journey. There is a directory on the Intuitive Eating website (see Resources, page 139) that you can use to find a provider. Many practitioners offer virtual support if you can't find someone in close proximity to you.

Progress Reflection Exercise

As you arrive toward the end of this book, take some time to reflect on how far you have come.

- What breakthroughs have you made regarding food and your body?

- In what ways have you experienced a shift in your behaviors around food or your emotional reaction to food?

- What fears do you continue to have regarding this journey?

- What has been challenging as you have attempted to shift your thinking around food and your body?

Putting It Together

In this chapter, we reviewed setting goals around food and movement that are gentle, supportive, and achievable. We reviewed the SMART approach to goal-setting as a way to find clarity on the path to achieving goals that are important to you. We also reviewed the importance of throwing the pass/fail mentality out the window in favor of allowing yourself to be human. Finally, we dove into keeping your healing journey moving forward, including working through negative thought patterns and enlisting support from others.

Let's review the exercises we have explored throughout the book:

- Contemplating your vision for your relationship with food

- Considering the factors that have contributed to your relationship with food today

- Thinking about the void dieting has filled in your life

- Curating your social media accounts to serve your healing journey

- Writing down how to counteract body-shaming environments

- Reflecting upon the ways in which your feelings about the appearance of your body have affected the way you have taken care of yourself

- Considering the factors that contribute to a desire to eat

- Exploring emotions that impact your desire to eat or not eat

- Writing down how to manage stressors in your life

- Practicing mindful eating

- Planning out meals and grocery shopping

- Engaging in a mood-boosting activity

- Setting SMART Goals

- Reframing achievement around food goals

I encourage you to continue to refer back to these exercises as you move forward on your journey of uncovering a new way to relate to food and your body.

Notes

Notes

Notes

Notes

Notes

Resources

Books

Anti-Diet, by Christy Harrison: Exposes the astounding harms of Diet Culture and explores alternative and much more effective ways of supporting your health

The Beauty Myth, by Naomi Wolf: An argument for the ways in which women of today are plagued by ever-increasing expectations around physical appearance that ultimately leave them just as restricted as they were in previous days of the homemaker wife

The Body Is Not an Apology, by Sonya Renee Taylor: A look at the ways systems of oppression thrive off of our inability to respect differences as well as a guide to finding self-love

Body Kindness, by Rebecca Scritchfield: A deeply compassionate and comprehensive take on the anti-diet approach that explores taking care of yourself in new ways

Body Respect, by Linda Bacon and Lucy Aphramor: A piece of work that builds on the *Health at Every Size* book, exploring more up-to-date research and continuing to argue for the ways that the dominant weight-centric model has failed us

Fat and Fertile, by Nicola Salmon: A guide for getting pregnant in a bigger body that challenges the widely held beliefs that you cannot

Fearing the Black Body, by Sabrina Strings: A compelling history that explores the connection between fat-phobia and racism

The Fuck It Diet, by Caroline Dooner: A comical account of the science behind why diets don't work, as well as a framework for healing your relationship with food

Health at Every Size, by Linda Bacon and Lucy Aphramor: A research-heavy piece of work that offers an in-depth look at the Health at Every Size model

Intuitive Eating, 4th Edition, by Evelyn Tribole and Elyse Resch: The latest edition of the original work that explained the Intuitive Eating framework

The Intuitive Eating Workbook, by Evelyn Tribole and Elyse Resch: A complement to the Intuitive Eating book that provides exercises to help readers explore their relationship with food on a deeper level to invoke healing

Landwhale, by Jes Baker: A look at life as a fat woman in our fat-phobic culture, including growing up fat and dating while fat

Things No One Will Tell Fat Girls, by Jes Baker: An invitation to reject the fat-phobic prejudice that continues to rage throughout our culture in favor of body positivity

You Have the Right to Remain Fat, by Virgie Tovar: A telling manifesto about rejecting Diet Culture and fat-phobia as well as starting to live your life now, no matter your size

Websites

BeautyRedefined.com: An organization committed to promoting positive body image in online spaces

HAESCommunity.com: A community of folks exploring Health at Every Size

IntuitiveEating.org: The Intuitive Eating website, including the community, research, and a directory of Certified Intuitive Eating Counselors

TheIntuitiveRD.com: Kirsten Ackerman's site that includes her various offerings for coaching and online courses

SizeDiversityAndHealth.org: Home to the organization that created the Health at Every Size model; includes resources as well as a directory of Health at Every Size–aligned practitioners

Podcasts

The Body Image Podcast with Corinne Dobbas: A podcast about body image and the process of making peace with our bodies

Body Image with Bri Podcast with Bri Campos: A podcast that aims to help listeners learn to love the bodies they are in

Body Kindness with Rebecca Scritchfield: Led by a Dietitian, a podcast that invites guests from various walks of life to discuss their paths toward better well-being

Dietitians Unplugged with Aaron Flores and Glenys Oyston: Led by two Registered Dietitians, a podcast that aims to help listeners improve their health, body image, and fitness without obsessing over the scale

Do No Harm with DeAun Nelson: A podcast dedicated to exploring the weight-inclusive model to health care as well as exposing the harms of the traditional weight-centric model

Food Psych with Christy Harrison: A podcast that talks with guests about their relationship with food and explores concepts of Intuitive Eating, Health at Every Size, and body liberation

Intuitive Bites Podcast with Kirsten Ackerman: Kirsten Ackerman's podcast, which aims to expose Diet Culture and explore topics including Intuitive Eating, Health at Every Size, and body liberation in short and sweet episodes

Love, Food with Julie Duffy Dillon: A podcast that explores our relationships with food through a unique take in which listeners write letters to specific foods

The Mindful Dietitian with Fiona Sutherland: A podcast that explores body inclusivity, Health at Every Size, the Non-Diet Approach, and mindfulness-based practice

Nutrition Matters with Paige Smathers: Led by a Registered Dietitian, a podcast that explores the Positive Nutrition approach to health

RD Real Talk with Heather Caplan: A podcast covering Intuitive Eating, anti-diet nutrition, eating disorder recovery, and sports nutrition

Unpacking Weight Science with Fiona Willer: A podcast that helps listeners understand weight-neutral research

References

Chapter 1

Bacon, Linda, and Lucy Aphramor. *Body Respect: What Conventional Health Books Get Wrong, Leave Out, and Just Plain Fail to Understand about Weight.* Dallas: BenBella Books, 2014.

Bacon, Linda, and Lucy Aphramor. "Weight Science: Evaluating the Evidence for a Paradigm Shift." *Nutrition Journal* 10, no. 9 (2011). doi.org/10.1186/1475-2891-10-9.

Center for Discovery. "What is an Eating Disorder?" Accessed February 7, 2020. CenterForDiscovery.com.

Tribole, Evelyn, and Elyse Resch. *Intuitive Eating: A Revolutionary Program That Works, 4th edition.* New York: St. Martin's Griffin, 2012.

Chapter 2

Association for Size Diversity and Health. "HAES Principles." Accessed February 7, 2020. SizeDiversityAndHealth.org /content.asp?id=152.

Bacon, Linda, and Lucy Aphramor. *Body Respect: What Conventional Health Books Get Wrong, Leave Out, and Just Plain Fail to Understand about Weight.* Dallas: BenBella Books, 2014.

Bacon, Linda, and Lucy Aphramor. "Weight Science: Evaluating the Evidence for a Paradigm Shift." *Nutrition Journal* 10, no. 9 (2011). doi.org/10.1186/1475-2891-10-9.

Chastain, Ragen. "What is Internalized Fatphobia?" Dances with Fat (blog). December 3, 2018. DancesWithFat .org/2018/12/03/what-is-internalized-fatphobia.

Dulloo, Abdul G., Jean Jacquet, and Jean-Pierre Montani. "How Dieting Makes Some Fatter: From a Perspective of Human Body Composition Autoregulation." *The Proceedings of the Nutrition Society* 71, no. 3 (August 2012): 379–89. doi.org/10.1017/S0029665112000225.

Gold, Tanya. "Obese Mannequins Are Selling Women a Dangerous Lie." *The Telegraph.* June 9, 2019. Telegraph .co.uk/women/life/obese-mannequins-selling-women -dangerous-lie.

Harrison, Christy. *Anti-Diet: Reclaim Your Time, Money, Well-Being, and Happiness Through Intuitive Eating.* New York: Little, Brown Spark, 2019.

Keys, Ancel, Austin Henschel, and Josef Brožek. *The Biology of Human Starvation.* Minneapolis: *University of Minnesota Press*, 1950.

LaRosa, John. "Top 9 Things to Know about the Weight Loss Industry." Market Research Blog. March 6, 2019. blog.MarketResearch.com/u.s.-weight-loss-industry -grows-to-72-billion

Louderback, Lew. "More People Should Be Fat." *The Saturday Evening Post.* November 4, 1967.

O'Hara, Lily, and Jane Taylor. "What's Wrong With the 'War on Obesity?' A Narrative Review of the Weight-Centered Health Paradigm and Development of the 3C Framework to Build Critical Competency for a Paradigm Shift." *Sage Open* 8, no. 2 (2018). doi.org/10.1177/2158244018772888.

Sobczak, Connie. *Embody: Learning to Love Your Unique Body (and Quiet That Critical Voice!)*. Nashville: Turner Publishing Company, 2014.

Technology Assessment Conference Panel. "Methods for Voluntary Weight Loss and Control." *Annals of Internal Medicine* 116, no. 11 (June 1992): 942–9. doi.org/10.7326/0003-4819-116-11-942.

Waaler, Hans T. "Height, Weight and Mortality. The Norwegian Experience." *Acta Medica Scandinavica* 215, no. S679 (1984). doi.org/10.1111/j.0954-6820.1984. tb12901.x.

Chapter 3

Dulloo, Abdul G., Jean Jacquet, and Jean-Pierre Montani. "How Dieting Makes Some Fatter: From a Perspective of Human Body Composition Autoregulation." *The Proceedings of the Nutrition Society* 71, no. 3 (August 2012): 379–89. doi.org/10.1017/S0029665112000225.

Satter, Ellyn. "Versions of Internally Regulated Eating." The Ellyn Satter Institute. Accessed February 7, 2020. EllynSatterInstitute.org/family-meals-focus/75-versions -of-internally-regulated-eating.

Chapter 4

Tribole, Evelyn, and Elyse Resch. *Intuitive Eating: A Revolutionary Program That Works, 4th edition.* New York: St. Martin's Griffin, 2012.

Chapter 5

Bacon, Linda, and Lucy Aphramor. *Body Respect: What Conventional Health Books Get Wrong, Leave Out, and Just Plain Fail to Understand about Weight.* Dallas: BenBella Books, 2014.

Indeed.com. "SMART Goals: Definition and Examples." March 11, 2020. Indeed.com/career-advice /career-development/smart-goals.

Index

Acknowledgments

Thank you to Callisto Media and to my editors Marisa Hines and Shabnam Sigman for supporting me in bringing the Intuitive Eating message to a wider audience.

I want to express my deepest gratitude to the fat activists whose work paved the way for the Intuitive Eating movement. I'm grateful to Evelyn Tribole and Elyse Resch for developing the Intuitive Eating framework, and to Christy Harrison, whose podcast, *Food Psych,* was my introduction to the concepts that have forever shifted my approaches to health and nutrition.

I want to acknowledge some amazing Health at Every Size and Intuitive Eating practitioners whose in-person support has been invaluable to me, including Brianna Campos, Julie Graham, Rachael Utstein, and Julia Werth.

I want to acknowledge the support of my family and friends who truly shared in my joy of writing this book, including Mary Bardwell, Phil Ackerman, Bette and Craig McVey, Luke and Carol Ackerman, Tyler McVey, Maggie McVey, Jake Morrisson, Tracie DeGonza, Annie Hall, and Mackenzie Riley.

And, last but not least, I want to thank my dogs, Sammy and Holly, for keeping me company during the long hours of writing.

About the Author

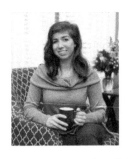 **Kirsten Ackerman** is an Anti-Diet, Fat-Positive Registered Dietitian, Certified Intuitive Eating Counselor, podcaster, and content creator. She obtained her BS in Nutrition Science from Russell Sage College and her MS in Applied Nutrition from Sage Graduate School, both located in Troy, NY.

Kirsten is dedicated to fighting Diet Culture and helping people heal their relationships with food and body. She resides in New Haven, CT, where she runs her virtual private practice for Intuitive Eating coaching. She is also the host of *Intuitive Bites Podcast* and sits on the board of the Connecticut Academy of Nutrition and Dietetics as the Events Coordinator. She has contributed to articles featured on POPSUGAR, *InStyle*, and more. Kirsten has been a guest on several podcasts, including *Food Psych* with Christy Harrison; *Love, Food* with Julie Duffy Dillon; and *Nutrition Matters* with Paige Smathers.

CPSIA information can be obtained
at www.ICGtesting.com
Printed in the USA
JSHW042038090620
6164JS00004B/11